CANCER ETIOLOGY, DIAGNOSIS AND TREATMENTS

SUN SAFETY FOR SCHOOLS AND YOUTH

SKIN CANCER PREVENTION GUIDANCE

CANCER ETIOLOGY, DIAGNOSIS AND TREATMENTS

Additional books in this series can be found on Nova's website under the Series tab.

Additional e-books in this series can be found on Nova's website under the e-book tab.

CANCER ETIOLOGY, DIAGNOSIS AND TREATMENTS

SUN SAFETY FOR SCHOOLS AND YOUTH

SKIN CANCER PREVENTION GUIDANCE

JARROD C. WALTON
EDITOR

nova publishers
New York

For permission to use material from this book please contact us:
Telephone 631-231-7269; Fax 631-231-8175
Web Site: http://www.novapublishers.com

Library of Congress Cataloging-in-Publication Data

ISBN: 978-1-63463-067-2

Published by Nova Science Publishers, Inc. † New York

CONTENTS

Preface		**vii**
Chapter 1	Guidelines for School Programs to Prevent Skin Cancer *Karen Glanz, Mona Saraiya and Howell Wechsler*	**1**
Chapter 2	Shade Planning for America's Schools *Centers for Disease Control and Prevention*	**43**
Chapter 3	Sun Safety for America's Youth Toolkit *Centers for Disease Control and Prevention*	**107**
Index		**153**

PREFACE

Skin cancer is the most common type of cancer in the United States. More than one half of a person's lifetime UV exposure occurs during childhood and adolescence because of more opportunities and time for exposure. Exposure to UV radiation during childhood plays a role in the future development of skin cancer. Studies indicate that protection from UV exposure during childhood and adolescence reduces the risk for skin cancer. These studies support the need to protect young persons from the sun beginning at an early age. School staff can play a major role in protecting children and adolescents from UV exposure and the future development of skin cancer by instituting policies, environmental changes, and educational programs that can reduce skin cancer risks among young persons. This book reviews scientific literature regarding the rates, trends, causes, and prevention of skin cancer and presents guidelines for schools to implement a comprehensive approach to preventing skin cancer.

Chapter 1 - Skin cancer is the most common type of cancer in the United States. Since 1973, new cases of the most serious form of skin cancer, melanoma, have increased approximately 150%. During the same period, deaths from melanoma have increased approximately 44%. Approximately 65%–90% of melanomas are caused by ultraviolet (UV) radiation. More than one half of a person's lifetime UV exposure occurs during childhood and adolescence because of more opportunities and time for exposure. Exposure to UV radiation during childhood plays a role in the future development of skin cancer. Persons with a history of ≥ 1 blistering sunburns during childhood or adolescence are two times as likely to develop melanoma than those who did not have such exposures. Studies indicate that protection from UV exposure during childhood and adolescence reduces the risk for skin cancer. These studies support the need to protect young persons from the sun beginning at an early age. School staff can play a major role in protecting children and adolescents from UV exposure and the future development of skin cancer by instituting policies, environmental changes, and educational programs that can reduce skin cancer risks among young persons.

This report reviews scientific literature regarding the rates, trends, causes, and prevention of skin cancer and presents guidelines for schools to implement a comprehensive approach to preventing skin cancer. Based on a review of research, theory, and current practice, these guidelines were developed by CDC in collaboration with specialists in dermatology, pediatrics, public health, and education; national, federal, state, and voluntary agencies; schools; and other organizations. Recommendations are included for schools to reduce skin cancer risks through policies; creation of physical, social, and organizational environments that facilitate protection from UV rays; education of young persons; professional development of staff; involvement of families; health services; and program evaluation.

Chapter 2 - In 2002, the Centers for Disease Control and Prevention (CDC) published the *Guidelines for School Programs to Prevent Skin Cancer*, which outlines steps that school communities can take to develop a comprehensive approach to reducing the risk for skin cancer among students, teachers, staff, and visitors. The guidelines include the following recommendations:

- Establish policies that reduce exposure to solar ultraviolet (UV) radiation.
- Provide and maintain physical and social environments that support sun safety.
- Provide opportunities for students to gain the knowledge, develop the attitudes, and practice the skills needed to prevent skin cancer.
- Involve family members in skin cancer prevention efforts.
- Provide pre-service and in-service skin cancer prevention education for school administrators, teachers, coaches, school nurses, and other professionals who work with students.
- Support sun-safety policies, sun-safe environments, and skin cancer prevention education with school health services.
- Evaluate the implementation of policies, environmental change, education, family involvement, professional development, and health services.

This manual has been created to support school communities in their implementation of the *Guidelines for School Programs to Prevent Skin Cancer* and, specifically, to help schools create and maintain a physical environment that supports sun safety by ensuring that school grounds have adequate shade.

Chapter 3 - Since 1998, the National Comprehensive Cancer Control Program (NCCCP) has provided funding and technical support to develop and implement comprehensive cancer control (CCC) plans to "reduce cancer incidence, morbidity, and mortality through prevention, early detection, treatment, rehabilitation and palliation." Currently the Centers for Disease Control and Prevention (CDC) Division of Cancer Prevention and Control (DCPC) "funds CCC programs in all 50 states, the District of Columbia, 7 tribes and tribal organization and 7 U.S. territories."

The CCC program in each state/tribe/territory/jurisdiction has a mandate to develop a plan that addresses a wide variety of cancer prevention and control priorities. This often includes skin cancer prevention. The Sun Safety for America's Youth Toolkit is designed as a resource for state/tribe/territory/ jurisdiction CCC programs interested in engaging schools and other education partners in sun safety efforts to reduce their state/tribe/territory/ jurisdiction's incidence of skin cancer. Since a majority of sun exposure occurs during childhood and early adulthood and key sun protective behaviors can most easily be established at this time, addressing sun safety for young people is an important cancer control objective.

There is a wide variety of sun safety programs, materials, and resources available to organizations interested in implementing sun safety efforts, many of which are described in this toolkit and the accompanying reference documents. This toolkit builds upon lessons learned from CDC's long history of sun safety and skin cancer prevention. In 2002, CDC released the *Guidelines for School Programs to Prevent Skin Cancer.* The Guidelines provide resources and suggestions for schools to improve sun safety practices in seven major areas: policy, environmental change, education, family involvement, professional development, health services, and evaluation. To foster implementation of these guidelines, DCPC, in partnership with the Division of Adolescent and School Health (DASH), made funds available to states with Coordinated School Health Programs (CSHPs) to conduct pilot skin cancer prevention activities. In 2003, through the Skin Cancer Priority Supplement to PA03004—Improving the Health, Education, and Well-Being of Young People through Coordinated School Health Programs—three states (Colorado, Michigan, and North Carolina) were awarded funds to pilot activities to address the school skin cancer guidelines. From late 2003 through early 2007, the Department of Education in each of the three funded states received funds to implement their pilot sun safety initiatives. Each state was required to develop an annual work plan that would guide their efforts to address CDC's skin cancer guidelines and develop a partnership with their state CCC program.

This toolkit draws from these efforts and is designed to provide CCC programs with resources and information that will help them to understand the burden of skin cancer within their state/tribe/territory/jurisdiction, assess current state/ tribe/territory/jurisdiction-level sun safety interest and activity, engage in implementation of sun safety efforts with schools and key education partners, and evaluate their efforts.

The toolkit consists of four key steps that will help CCC programs move through a logical process for engaging and implementing sun safety efforts for young people:

- Step I: Identify and Recruit Sun Safety Partners
- Step II: Assess and Understand Sun Safety Needs and Resources in Your State/Tribe/Territory/Jurisdiction
- Step III: Plan and Implement Sun Safety Activities
- Step IV: Evaluate Sun Safety Efforts

Step I describes the numerous organizations and individuals CCC programs may want to engage in sun safety planning and implementation. These partners represent both state/tribe/territory/jurisdiction and local organizations that can play an important role in reaching schools and young people to implement and enhance effective sun safety strategies.

Step II provides recommendations for understanding the current state skin cancer burden and how to utilize that information to inform the development and targeting of sun safety efforts. To understand the current level of sun safety activity within the state/tribe/territory/jurisdiction, recommendations and resources are provided for conducting a sun safety program and resource inventory at the state/tribe/territory/jurisdiction level. Resources are also provided to help your CCC program understand the current legal and/or policy issues related to sun safety and how sun safety may already be integrated into existing school resources and tools.

Step III outlines a process for conducting a Strengths, Weaknesses, Opportunities and Threats (SWOT) analysis related to implementation of sun safety activities. Recommendations and resources on selection of sun safety activities are provided as well as examples of activities implemented using the *CDC Guidelines for School Programs to Prevent Skin Cancer*.

Step IV highlights the importance of evaluation of state/tribe/territory/jurisdiction sun safety efforts and offers some examples of how to evaluate sun safety efforts locally and at the state/tribe/territory/jurisdiction level. We also provide suggestions for modification of state surveillance systems.

Within each step, we provide examples from state sun safety efforts to help CCC programs understand how these recommendations, tools, and resources have been utilized by other states.

The toolkit also includes an extensive sun safety resource list, which highlights potential sun safety partners at the state/tribe/territory/jurisdiction and national levels, and other sun safety programs and materials that are currently available.

In: Sun Safety for Schools and Youth
Editor: Jarrod C. Walton

ISBN: 978-1-63463-067-2

Chapter 1

GUIDELINES FOR SCHOOL PROGRAMS TO PREVENT SKIN CANCER*

Karen Glanz, Mona Saraiya and Howell Wechsler

SUMMARY

Skin cancer is the most common type of cancer in the United States. Since 1973, new cases of the most serious form of skin cancer, melanoma, have increased approximately 150%. During the same period, deaths from melanoma have increased approximately 44%. Approximately 65%–90% of melanomas are caused by ultraviolet (UV) radiation. More than one half of a person's lifetime UV exposure occurs during childhood and adolescence because of more opportunities and time for exposure. Exposure to UV radiation during childhood plays a role in the future development of skin cancer. Persons with a history of ≥1 blistering sunburns during childhood or adolescence are two times as likely to develop melanoma than those who did not have such exposures. Studies indicate that protection from UV exposure during childhood and adolescence reduces the risk for skin cancer. These studies support the need to protect young persons from the sun beginning at an early age. School staff can play a major role in protecting children and adolescents from UV exposure and the future development of skin cancer by

* This is an edited, reformatted and augmented version of Morbidity and Mortality Weekly Report, April 26, 2002, Vol. 51, No. RR-4, issued by the Centers for Disease Control and Prevention.

instituting policies, environmental changes, and educational programs that can reduce skin cancer risks among young persons.

This report reviews scientific literature regarding the rates, trends, causes, and prevention of skin cancer and presents guidelines for schools to implement a comprehensive approach to preventing skin cancer. Based on a review of research, theory, and current practice, these guidelines were developed by CDC in collaboration with specialists in dermatology, pediatrics, public health, and education; national, federal, state, and voluntary agencies; schools; and other organizations. Recommendations are included for schools to reduce skin cancer risks through policies; creation of physical, social, and organizational environments that facilitate protection from UV rays; education of young persons; professional development of staff; involvement of families; health services; and program evaluation.

INTRODUCTION

Skin cancer is the most common type of cancer in the United States [1]. Since 1973, the number of new cases of melanoma, the skin cancer with the highest risk for mortality and one of the most common cancers among young adults, has increased. The incidence of melanoma has increased 150%, and melanoma mortality rates have increased by 44% [1]. Because a substantial percentage of lifetime sun exposure occurs before age 20 years [2,3] and because ultraviolet (UV) radiation exposure during childhood and adolescence plays an important role in the development of skin cancer [2,4], preventive behaviors can yield the most positive effects, if they are initiated early and established as healthy and consistent patterns throughout life. Children spend several hours at school on most weekdays, and some of that time is spent in outdoor activities. Schools, therefore, are in a position to teach and model healthy behaviors, and they can use health education activities involving families to encourage sun-safe behaviors at home. Thus, schools can play a vital role in preventing skin cancer.

This report is one of a series of guidelines produced by CDC to help schools improve the health of young persons by promoting behaviors to prevent the leading causes of illness and death [5–8]. The primary audience for this report includes state and local health and educational agencies and nongovernmental organizations concerned with improving the health of U.S. students. These agencies and organizations can translate the information in this report into materials and training programs for their constituents. In addition, CDC will develop and disseminate materials to help schools and school districts implement the guidelines. At the local level, teachers and other school personnel, community recreation program personnel, health service providers, community leaders, policymakers, and parents may use these guidelines and complementary materials to plan and implement skin cancer prevention policies and programs. In addition, faculty at institutions of higher education may use these guidelines to train professionals in education, public health, sports and recreation, school psychology, nursing, medicine, and other appropriate disciplines.

Although these skin cancer prevention guidelines are intended for schools, they can also guide child care facilities and other organizations that provide opportunities for children and adolescents to spend time in outdoor settings (e.g., camps; sports fields; playgrounds; swimming, tennis, and boating clubs; farms; and recreation and park facilities). These guidelines address children and adolescents of primary-and secondary-school age (approximately 5–18 years). The recommendations are based on scientific evidence, medical and behavioral knowledge, and consensus among specialists in education and skin cancer prevention. In 2003, CDC will publish a chapter on cancer in its *Community Guide to Preventive Services* [9], which will summarize information regarding the effectiveness of community-based interventions geared to-ward preventing skin cancer.

School-based programs can play an important role in achieving the following national Health Objectives for the Year 2010 related to skin cancer prevention: 1) increase the proportion of persons who use at least one of the following protective measures that might reduce the risk for skin cancer: avoid the sun between 10 a.m. and 4 p.m., wear sun-protective clothing when exposed to the sun, use sunscreen with a sun-protection factor (SPF) ≥15, and avoid artificial sources of UV light; and 2) reduce deaths from melanoma to <2.5 per 100,000 persons [10].

Burden of Skin Cancer

Skin cancer is the most common type of cancer in the United States [11]. The two most common kinds of skin cancer — basal cell carcinoma and squamous cell carcinoma — are highly curable. However, melanoma, the third most common type of skin cancer and one of the most common cancers among young adults, is more dangerous. In 2001, approximately 1.3 million new cases of basal cell or squamous cell carcinoma were diagnosed with approximately 2,000 deaths from basal cell and squamous cell carcinoma combined. Melanoma, by contrast, will be diagnosed in 53,600 persons and will account for 7,400 deaths, more than three fourths of all skin cancer deaths [12].

Basal cell carcinoma, which accounts for 75% of all skin cancers [11], rarely metastasizes to other organs. Squamous cell carcinoma, which accounts for 20% of all skin cancers, has a higher likelihood of spreading to the lymph nodes and internal organs and causing death [13], but these outcomes are also rare. Melanoma is nearly always curable in its early stages, but it is most likely to spread to other parts of the body if detected late. Melanoma most often appears on the trunk of men and the lower legs of women, although it also might be found on the head, neck, or elsewhere [14,15].

In the United States, diagnoses of new melanomas are increasing, whereas diagnoses of the majority of other cancers are decreasing [16]. Since 1973, the annual incidence rate for melanoma (new cases diagnosed per 100,000 persons) has more than doubled, from 5.7 cases per 100,000 in that year to 14.3 per 100,000 in 1998 [1] (Figure). The rapid increase in annual incidence rates is likely a result of several factors, including increased exposure to UV radiation and possibly earlier detection of melanoma [17]. Since 1973, annual deaths per 100,000 persons from melanoma have increased by approximately 44%, from 1.6 to 2.3 (Figure). However, over the course of the 1990s, mortality rates have remained stable, particularly among women (16,18–19]. Although doctors must report other types of cancer (including melanomas) to cancer registries, they are not required to report squamous or basal cell cancer, which makes tracking trends in the incidence of these two cancers difficult. However, death rates for basal cell and squamous cell carcinoma have remained stable [12].

Risk Factors for Skin Cancer

Excessive Exposure to UV Radiation

Skin cancer is largely preventable by limiting exposure to the primary source of UV radiation, sunlight. Sunlamps and tanning beds are other sources. Persons with high levels of exposure to UV radiation are at an increased risk for all three major forms of skin cancer. Approximately 65%–90% of melanomas are caused by UV exposure [20]. The epidemiology implicating UV exposure as a cause of melanoma is further supported by biologic evidence that damage caused by UV radiation, particularly damage to DNA, plays a central role in the development of melanoma [4]. Total UV exposure depends on the intensity of the light, duration of skin exposure, and whether the skin was protected by sun-protective clothing and sunscreen. Severe, blistering sunburns are associated with an increased risk for both melanoma and basal cell carcinoma. For these cancers, intermittent intense exposures seem to carry higher risk than do lower level, chronic, or cumulative exposures, even if the total UV dose is the same. In contrast, the risk for squamous cell carcinoma is strongly associated with chronic UV exposure but not with intermittent exposure.

The two most important types of UV radiation, UV-A and UV-B radiation, have both been linked to the development of skin cancer. UV-A rays are not absorbed by the ozone layer, penetrate deeply into the skin, and cause premature aging and possibly suppression of the immune system [4,21,22]. Up to 90% of the visible changes commonly attributable to aging are caused by sun exposure. UV-B rays, which are partially absorbed by the ozone layer, tan and sometimes burn the skin. UV-B radiation has been linked to the development of cataracts [23–25] and skin cancer. Recommended skin cancer prevention measures protect against both UV-A and UV-B radiation.

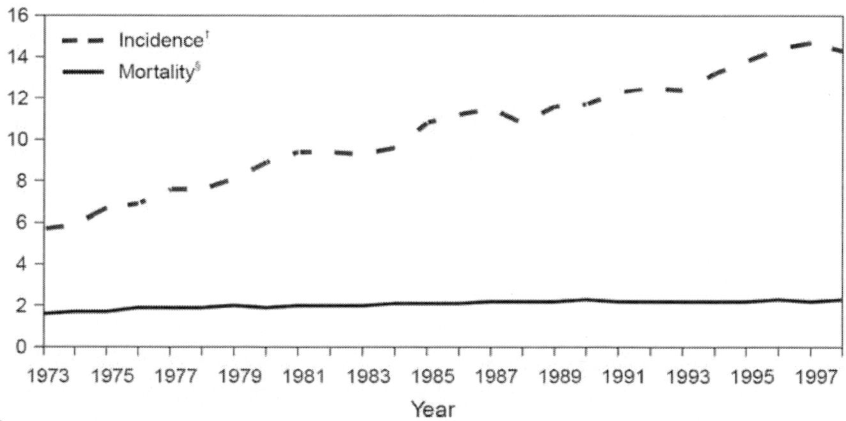

* Rate is age-adjusted to 1970 U.S. population.

† 1973 Incidence rate: 5.7 per 100,000 persons; 1998 incidence rate: 14.3 per 100,000.

§ 1973 Mortality rate: 1.6 per 100,000; 1998 mortality rate: 2.3 per 100,000.

Source: Cancer Statistics Review, 1973–1998.

Figure. Melanoma of the skin (invasive): SEER incidence and U.S. mortality rates*, 1973–1998.

Childhood and Adolescent UV Exposure

Exposure to UV radiation during childhood and adolescence plays a role in the future development of both melanoma and basal cell cancer [26–32]. For example, the risk for developing melanoma is related strongly to a history of $\geq$1 sunburns (an indicator of intense UV exposure) in childhood or adolescence [27,28,33,34). Similarly, sunburns during these periods have been demonstrated to increase the risk for basal cell carcinoma [30,*31*].

Childhood is the most important time for developing moles, which is an important risk factor for skin cancer. Sun exposure in childhood might increase the risk for melanoma by increasing the number of moles [*33*]. A study supports the use of sun protection during childhood to reduce the risk for melanoma in adulthood [35].

Children and adolescents have more opportunities and time than adults to be exposed to sunlight [36–38] and thus more opportunities for development of skin cancer [4,39,40]. More than one half of a person's lifetime UV exposure occurs during childhood and adolescence [3,41].

Skin Color and Ethnicity

Although anyone can get skin cancer, persons with certain characteristics are particularly at risk. For example, the incidence of melanoma among whites is approximately 20 times higher than among blacks [1]. Hispanics appear to be at less risk for melanoma than whites; a study conducted in Los Angeles, California, indicated that the incidence rates for Hispanics were 2–3 per 100,000, whereas the rate for non-Hispanic whites was 11 per 100,000 [42]. For basal cell and squamous cell carcinoma, rates among blacks are 1/80 of the rates among whites [43].

The ethnic differences in observed rates are attributable mostly to skin color. The color of the skin is determined by the amount of melanin produced by melanocytes, which also protect the skin from the damage produced by UV radiation. Although darkly pigmented persons develop skin cancer on sun-exposed sites at lower rates than lightly pigmented persons, UV exposure increases their risk for developing skin cancer [44]. The risk for skin cancer is higher among persons who sunburn readily and tan poorly [45], namely those with red or blond hair, and fair skin that freckles or burns easily [14,46,47].

Moles

The most measurable predictors of melanoma are having large numbers and unusual types of moles (nevi) [48,49]. Usually not present at birth, moles begin appearing during childhood and adolescence and are associated with sun exposure. Most moles are harmless but some undergo abnormal changes and become melanomas. A changing mole, particularly in an adult, is often indicative of the development of melanoma [45].

Family History

The risk for melanoma increases if a person has ≥1 first-degree relatives (i.e., mother, father, brother, and sister) with the disease. Depending on the number of affected relatives, the risk can be up to eight times that of persons without a family history of melanoma. Nonetheless, only approximately 10% of all persons with melanoma have a family history of melanoma [45,50].

Age

The incidence of skin cancer increases exponentially with age because older persons have had more opportunities to be exposed to UV radiation and they have diminished capacity to repair the damage from UV radiation [4,14,43]. Approximately one half of all melanomas occur in persons aged <50 years. Melanoma is one of the most common cancers found in persons aged <30 years [14]; it is the most common cancer occurring among persons in the 25–29 age group and the third most common in the 20–24 age group [51].

Environmental Factors Affecting UV Radiation

Environmental factors that increase the amount of UV radiation exposure received by humans include a latitude closer to the equator; higher altitude; light cloud coverage (allows 80% of UV rays to go through the clouds); the presence of materials that reflect the sun (e.g. pavement, water, snow, and sand); being outside near noontime (UV-B radiation is highest in the middle of the day and varies more by time of day than does UV-A); and being outside during the spring or summer [21,52]. Ozone depletion could potentially increase levels of solar radiation at the earth's surface [53,54].

Artificial UV Radiation

In 2000, the National Institute of Environmental Health Sciences concluded that sunlamps and tanning beds are carcinogenic [55]. Although limited, epidemiologic evidence suggests that a causal relation exists between artificial UV radiation and melanoma [55,56]. The type and amount of UV radiation emitted from some sunbeds appear to be similar to that of noontime summer sun, and in some cases, the amount is even higher than the sun would emit [57]. Artificial UV radiation can substantially damage the skin (i.e., cause sunburn) and has been linked to ocular melanoma [52,58]. Sunlamps and tanning beds should be avoided.

Protective Behaviors

Options for skin cancer prevention (Box 1) include limiting or minimizing exposure to the sun during peak hours (10 a.m.–4 p.m.), especially the 1-hour period closest to the noon hour (11 a.m.–1:00 p.m. when the UV rays are the strongest), wearing sun-protective clothing, using sunscreens that have UV-A and UV-B protection, and avoiding sunlamps and tanning beds. Most medical and cancer organizations advocate the use of similar skin cancer prevention measures [59]. The American Cancer Society [60], the American Academy of Dermatology [61,62], the American Academy of Pediatrics [63], the American Medical Association [64], and the National Cancer Institute [65] all recommend patient education on UV radiation avoidance and sunscreen use. The third U.S. Preventive Services Task Force is revising their guidelines on provider counseling for skin cancer prevention and sunscreen use.

Box 1. Skin Cancer Protective Behaviors

- Minimize exposure to the sun during peak hours (10 a.m.–4 p.m.).
- Seek shade from the midday sun (10 a.m.– 4 p.m.).
- Wear clothing, hats, and sunglasses that protect the skin.
- Use a broad-spectrum sunscreen (UV-A and UV-B protection) with a sun-protection factor of ≥15.
- Avoid sunlamps and tanning beds.

Avoiding the Sun and Wearing Proper Clothing and Sunglasses

Some forms of protection (e.g., avoiding the sun, seeking shade, and wearing sun-protective clothing) are the first approach toward preventing skin cancer. One study has demonstrated that wearing sun-protective clothing can decrease the number of moles [66]; another study demonstrated that the protective effect of clothing depends primarily on the construction of the fabric (a tighter weave permits less UV radiation to reach the skin) [67]. Other important factors include fiber type (natural cotton or Lycra™ transmits less UV radiation than bleached cotton) and color (darker colors transmit less UV radiation); additional factors include whether the fabric is wet or stretched (transmission of UV radiation increases as the fabric becomes more wet and stretched) [68]. Wide-brimmed hats (>3-inch brim) and Legionnaire hats (baseball type of hat with attached ear and neck flaps) provide the best protection for the head, ears, nose, and cheeks [69]. In 2001, the Federal Trade Commission and the Consumer Safety Product Commission assisted in the development of voluntary industry standards in the United States for rating the UV protective value of different types of clothing and of shade structures [70]. These standards should help the public make informed decisions concerning protection against UV radiation [68,71].

Sunglasses protect the eyes and surrounding areas from UV damage and skin cancer. Although no federal regulations exist for sunglasses, the American Academy of Ophthalmology recommends that sunglasses block 99% of UV-A and UV-B radiation. A chemical coating applied to the surface of the lens is the protective mechanism; protection does not correlate with the color or darkness of the lens [72]. Sunglasses can reduce UV radiation exposure to the eye by 80%, and when combined with a wide-brimmed hat or Legionnaire hat, UV exposure to the face is reduced by 65% [73].

Shade structures and trees can reduce direct UV radiation, but the protection offered is dependent on the direct and indirect UV radiation from the surrounding surface (e.g., sand and concrete) [74,75]. For example, umbrellas with more overhang provide more UV protection than those with less overhang.

Sunscreens

Sunscreens are an important adjunct to other types of protection against UV exposure. Using sunscreen is one of the most commonly practiced behaviors for preventing skin cancer.

During the previous decade, new studies have contributed to an increased understanding of the role of sunscreen in possibly preventing skin cancer. The U.S. Preventive Services Task Force is revising their recommendations on sunscreen use, but the International Agency for Research on Cancer has concluded that topical use of sunscreens probably prevents squamous cell carcinoma of the skin. The group drew no conclusions regarding whether the use of sunscreens reduces the incidence of basal cell carcinoma or melanoma [76] (Appendix A).

Clinical trials have demonstrated that sunscreens are effective in reducing the incidence of actinic keratoses, the precursors to squamous cell carcinoma [77,78]. One randomized clinical trial demonstrated that sunscreens are effective in reducing squamous cell carcinoma itself [79]. Another randomized trial demonstrated that, among children who are at high risk for developing melanoma, sunscreens are effective in reducing moles, the precursors and strongest risk factor for melanoma [80]. Unfortunately, many persons use sunscreens if they intend to stay out in the sun longer, and they reduce the use of other forms of sun protection (e.g., clothing or hats), thereby, acquiring the same or even a higher amount of UV radiation exposure than they would have obtained with a shorter stay and no sunscreen [22,76,81].

The guidelines in this report recommend 1) using various methods (e.g., avoiding the sun, seeking shade, or wearing protective clothing) that reduce exposure to the full spectrum of UV radiation as the first line of protection against skin cancer and 2) using sunscreen as a complementary measure. In some instances, sunscreens might be the only responsible option. However, to be effective, sunscreens must be applied correctly (Appendix B). For example, users should apply sunscreen and allow it to dry before going outdoors and getting any UV exposure [82,83]. Similarly, users should reapply sunscreen after leaving the water, sweating, or drying off with a towel. Use of insufficient quantities of sunscreen [84,85] or use of a sunscreen with insufficient protection are other concerns. Manufacturers determine the SPF (a measure of protection from only UV-B radiation) by applying an adequate amount of sunscreen (1–2 ounces) on humans and testing under artificial light, which is usually not as strong as natural light [86]. No government standards measure how much protection sunscreens provide against UV-A rays.

Few studies have been conducted on sunscreens, despite their widespread use, which make it difficult to estimate the prevalence of allergies to sunscreens. Skin irritation, rather than an actual allergic reaction, is one of the more commonly reported adverse events [87]. Because the majority of the commercially available sunscreens are a combination of agents from various chemical groups, persons who might experience adverse effects should be aware of the active ingredients and try sunscreens with different ingredients. In previous years, the most commonly reported allergen was para-aminobenzoic acid (PABA) (rarely used today), whereas the current two most frequently cited allergens are benzophenone-3 and dibenzoyl methanes [22].

Prevalence of Behavioral Risk Factors, Sun-Safe Behaviors, and Attitudes Related to Sun Safety

In the United States, sunbathing and tanning habits were established during the early to mid-1900s [88,89], most likely reflecting the increased availability of leisure time and fashion trends promoting tanned skin [89,90]. In the late 1970s, the majority of the population had little knowledge concerning their personal susceptibility to skin cancer and believed that tanning enhanced appearance and was associated with better health [91]. More recent reports indicate that many Americans feel healthier with a tan and believe that suntanned skin is more attractive [36,92,93].

In 1992, 53% of U.S. adults were "very likely" to protect themselves from the sun by practicing at least one protective behavior (using sunscreen, seeking shade, or wearing sunprotective clothing) [94]. Among white adults, approximately one third used sunscreen (32%), sought shade (30%), and wore protective clothing (28%). Among black adults, 45% sought shade, 28% wore sun-protective clothing, and 9% used sunscreen [95]. Sun-protective behaviors were more common among the more sun sensitive, females, and older age groups among both whites and blacks.

Sun-safety behaviors might be most difficult to change among preadolescents and adolescents [96]. Teenagers spend a substantial amount of time outdoors, especially on weekends and during the summer [97,98]. Many teenagers believe that a tan is desirable [92]; only teenagers who know persons with skin cancer or who perceive an increased personal susceptibility to skin cancer are more likely to use sunscreen [98]. However, teenagers who practice skin cancer prevention tend to only use sunscreen and to use it infrequently, inconsistently, and incorrectly [97,98]. Girls tend to use sunscreen more than boys, but they also use tanning beds more frequently [97–101].

Sunscreen use by children is correlated positively with use by their parents [87,102]. Some parents know the risks of skin cancer but do not realize that children are at risk [103,104]. Some parents believe that a suntan is a sign of good health; others use sunscreen on their children as their only or preferred skin cancer prevention measure [36,99,105–107], even though other measures (e.g., using shade structures and wearing sunprotective clothing) are available. Sometimes parents apply sunscreen on their children incorrectly and inconsistently [22] (e.g., only after a child has experienced a painful sunburn) [97,108].

Concerns Regarding Promoting Protection from UV Radiation

Sun-safety measures should not reduce student participation in physical activity. Regular physical activity reduces morbidity and mortality for multiple chronic diseases. Promoting lifelong physical activity in schools is a critically important public health and educational priority [8]. Schools might find it difficult to avoid scheduling outdoor physical activity programs around the midday hours. These schools can focus their efforts on other sun-safety measures (e.g., seeking shade; and wearing a hat, protective clothing, or sunscreen), which can be implemented without compromising physical activity while gradually making feasible scheduling changes.

In addition, because UV radiation plays a role in the synthesis of vitamin D, the limitation of UV exposure might be of some concern. This limitation might lead to a decrease in levels of vitamin D and increase the likelihood that rickets, a disorder involving a weakening of the bones, will develop in susceptible infants and children. However, the average age for presentation of rickets is 18 months, and the age groups of concern are typically infants and toddlers, not school-aged children between 5 and 18 years. Although the major source of vitamin D is through skin exposure to sunlight, supplementing the diet with foods (e.g., flesh of fatty fish, eggs from hens fed vitamin D, and vitamin D-fortified milk and breakfast cereal) can provide enough vitamin D to meet adequate intake requirements [109,110]. The American Academy of Pediatrics [111] recommends vitamin D supplementation for breast-fed infants whose mothers are vitamin D deficient or for infants who are not exposed to adequate sunlight. Infants consuming at least 500ml of vitamin D-fortified formula per day and older children consuming at least 16 ounces of vitamin D-fortified milk per day will meet the adequate intake of vitamin D.

Guidelines for School Programs to Prevent Skin Cancer

Schools as Settings for Skin Cancer Prevention Efforts

Epidemiologic data suggest that several skin cancers can be prevented if children and adolescents are protected from UV radiation [26–32]. Schools can participate in reducing exposure of young persons to UV radiation from the sun during school-related activities by offering education and skill-building activities to reinforce the development of healthful behaviors. School-based efforts to prevent skin cancer can be more effective in the framework of a coordinated school health program [112,113] that includes family and community participation [114] and builds on the context and current practices in the school and community. Coordinated school health programs aim to create and support environments where young persons can gain the knowledge, attitudes, and skills required to make and maintain healthy choices and habits. These programs integrate health education, a healthy school environment, physical education, nutrition services, health services, mental health and counseling services, health promotion programs for faculty and staff, and efforts to integrate school activities with family and community life [113].

Being aware of existing practices for sun exposure and sun protection among teachers, staff, and students might help define gaps in optimal sun-safety practices. Careful observations for a few days might also provide important information concerning students' use of shade areas and sunscreen at recess or lunch time, and staff's use of hats, shirts, and sunglasses. Discussions with students and staff who practice sun-safe behaviors might prove useful in planning and improving implementation of sun-safety practices.

Skin cancer prevention measures vary in both their ease of adoption and relevance. Schools should not allow an "all or nothing" approach to undermine the effectiveness of their skin cancer prevention efforts. For sun-safety protection, a shortsleeve shirt and cap might be better than no hat and a sleeveless top. Being flexible is important while moving in the direction of optimal skin cancer prevention environments, policies, and programs.

SKIN CANCER PREVENTION GUIDELINES

These guidelines provide recommendations for skin cancer prevention activities within a coordinated school health program. In addition, these guidelines are based on scientific literature, national policy documents, current practice, and theories and principles of health behavioral change [115]. Schools and community organizations can work together to develop plans that are relevant and achievable. Sustained support from school staff, students, communities, state and local education and health agencies, families, institutions of higher education, and national organizations are necessary to ensure the effectiveness of school skin cancer prevention activities [116].

In this report, seven broad guidelines are included that school programs can use to reduce the risk for skin cancer among students: 1) policy, 2) environmental change, 3) education, 4) families, 5) professional development, 6) health services, and 7) evaluation (Box 2). Each guideline includes suggestions regarding key elements, steps for implementation, and realistic expectations for change.

Box 2. Recommendations for Skin Cancer Prevention in Schools

1. Establish **policies** that reduce exposure to ultraviolet radiation.
2. Provide an **environment** that supports sun-safety practices.
3. Provide health **education** to teach students the knowledge, attitudes, and behavioral skills they need to prevent skin cancer.
4. Involve **family** members in skin cancer prevention efforts.
5. Include skin cancer prevention with **professional development** of staff (e.g., preservice and in-service education).
6. Complement and support skin cancer prevention with school **health services**.
7. Periodically **evaluate** whether schools are implementing the guidelines on policies, environmental change, education, families, professional development, and health services.

- **Guideline 1: Policy** — Establish policies that reduce exposure to UV radiation.
- **Guideline 2: Environmental change** — Provide and maintain physical and social environments that support sun safety and that are consistent with the development of other healthful habits.
- **Guideline 3: Education** — Provide health education to teach students the knowledge, attitudes, and behavioral skills they need to prevent skin cancer. The education should be age-appropriate and linked to opportunities for practicing sun-safety behaviors.
- **Guideline 4: Family Involvement** — Involve family members in skin cancer prevention efforts.
- **Guideline 5: Professional development** — Include skin cancer prevention knowledge and skills in preservice and in-service education for school administrators, teachers, physical education teachers and coaches, school nurses, and others who work with students.
- **Guideline 6: Health services** — Complement and support skin cancer prevention education and sun-safety environments and policies with school health services.
- **Guideline 7: Evaluation** — Periodically evaluate whether schools are implementing the guidelines on policies, environmental change, education, families, professional development, and health services.

The recommendations represent the state-of-the-science in school-based skin cancer prevention. However, every recommendation is not appropriate or feasible for every school to implement nor should any school be expected to implement all recommendations. Schools should determine which recommendations have the highest priority based on the needs of the school and available resources. As more resources become available, schools could implement additional recommendations to support a coordinated approach to preventing skin cancer.

Guideline 1: Policy — Establish Policies that Reduce Exposure to UV Radiation

Policies can provide sun protection for all persons in a defined population (e.g., a school), not just those who are most motivated [117]. In addition, policies can involve formal organizational rules and standards or legal requirements and restrictions related to skin cancer prevention measures. Policies may be developed by a school, school board, or by other legal entities (e.g., municipal, state, and federal governments). To be effective, policies need to be communicated to school personnel, announced to affected constituents (e.g., students and their parents), managed and implemented, enforced and monitored, and reviewed periodically [118,119].

Before establishing healthy skin cancer prevention policies, identify any existing policies that might deter skin cancer prevention. These existing policies might include outdoor activity schedules, prohibitions on wearing sunglasses or caps and hats at school, and rules that limit the use or provision of sunscreen at school (e.g., requiring parental permission, defining sunscreen as "medicine", and restricting teachers from applying sunscreen on children). California enacted a law (effective January 2002) that requires their schools to allow students, when outdoors, to w ear school-site approved sun-protective hats and clothing. This legislation was deemed necessary because several school districts had banned hats because some styles or colors are connected with gang affiliation.

An effectively crafted skin cancer prevention policy provides a framework for implementing the other six guidelines. The policy demonstrates institutional commitment and guides school and community groups in planning, implementing, and evaluating skin cancer prevention activities. Such a policy creates a supportive environment for students to learn about and adopt sun-protection practices. Although a comprehensive policy is preferable, more limited policies addressing certain aspects of skin cancer prevention also can be useful.

Developing the Policy or Policies

Skin cancer prevention can be part of a larger school health policy. Although policies might be initiated by a person or small group, the most effective policies are developed with input from all relevant constituents. In schools, the constituents include students, teachers, parents, administrators, coaches, school nurses, health educators and other relevant personnel as well as community leaders and residents. Schools can also work with community partners (e.g., recreation and parks departments, health departments, after-school programs, camps, families, and youth advocacy groups) and others who organize outdoor activities for youth.

Policies require time for development and implementation and might not be as visible as educational programs [120]. Increased effort in the early stages of policy development might result in increased adoption [121]. In Australia, health and cancer prevention specialists developed a sun-protection policy kit for schools and a related staff development module [*120*]. Elementary schools were twice as likely to formally adopt a comprehensive sun-protection policy if they also received the staff development module (44% [kit and module] versus 21% [kit only]). However, few high schools adopted policies whether they received just the kit or the kit and the module (11% and 6%, respectively) [120]. Policy development requires a longterm commitment and sustained efforts and cooperation among all concerned parties.

Policy Options

Components of skin cancer prevention policies for a school or community to consider include 1) statement of purpose and goals; 2) schedule and physical environment policies; 3) policies related to personal protective clothing and sunglasses; 4) sunscreen policies; 5) education policies; 6) policies on outreach to families; and 7) policies on resource allocation and evaluation. When implementing a comprehensive policy (which would include all of these components) is not feasible, schools can start with some of these components and add others over time.

Policy 1: Statement of Purpose and Goals. Policies usually begin with a statement of purpose and goals that establish sun safety as a priority and highlight the importance of skin cancer prevention. In addition, the statement can 1) describe the influence of childhood sun exposure on the risk for developing skin cancer later in life; 2) identify actions that persons and institutions can take to reduce the risk for skin cancer; 3) highlight the importance of establishing a physical, social, and organizational environment that supports skin cancer prevention; and 4) specify dedicated financial and human resources for skin cancer prevention and for the other policy options described here.

Policy 2: Schedule and Structure Policies. Policies can provide the basis for across-the-board reduction of UV radiation exposure for children and adults in schools and communities by establishing 1) rules that encourage the scheduling of outdoor activities (including athletic and sporting events) during times when the sun is not at its peak intensity and 2) building and grounds codes to increase the availability of shade in frequently used outdoor spaces.

Eliminating the scheduling of outdoor activities during peak sun hours will be difficult, if not impossible, for many schools to do. For these schools, the best strategy might be to work toward a gradual shift in scheduling. School board policies could require architects to design new school buildings with adequate shade coverage adjacent to play and sports fields. Play and sports fields can be reviewed for existing and potential shade. School and community organization staff could evaluate frequently used spaces in the community for their UV protection status and add signs, reminders, or prompts to encourage sun safety. Finally, volunteer, business, health department, and political support can be secured by school and community organization staff to generate resources for improving the sun-safety environment, especially for providing sunscreen and shade.

Policy 3: Policies for Personal Protective Clothing and Sunglasses. Schools can develop policies that encourage or require students to wear protective clothing, hats, and sunglasses to prevent excessive sun exposure. These measures could be employed during physical education classes, recess, field trips, outdoor sports or band events, and camping or field trips. Some schools, especially in Australia, have a "no hat/no play" policy stating that students cannot play outdoors if they are not wearing hats [119]. Related policy initiatives could require the use of athletic, band, and physical education uniforms that reduce or minimize excessive sun exposure (e.g., long sleeves and broad-brimmed hats). Strategies that can be implemented to promote the adoption of these policies include gradually phasing-in new policies that involve students and sports teams designing new uniforms, securing business sponsorship for sun-safe uniforms, and conducting discussions that promote the use of hats and sunglasses.

Some schools might have policies that prohibit or discourage students and staff from wearing hats and sunglasses on school grounds (e.g., because they are associated with contraband or gang-related items). Possible transmission of head lice among younger children who share hats might also be a concern; however, policies can be implemented that address these concerns (e.g., prohibiting both sharing hats and wearing gang-related symbols).

Policy 4: Sunscreen Policies. Policies on sunscreen use at school or for after-school activities can range from encouraging parents to include sunscreen in required school-supply kits, using permission slips for students to be able to apply sunscreen at school [122], and establishing a sunscreen use routine before going outside. Policies also might require teachers and coaches to use sunscreen for outside activities and require that sunscreen be provided at official school-sponsored events that occur during midday. Necessary steps that might be implemented include modifying existing policies that restrict school-based sunscreen application [123], seeking support for purchasing sunscreen supplies, and supervising sunscreen use.

Policy 5: Education Policies. The ideal education policy should support planned and sequential health education to provide students with the knowledge, attitudes, and behavioral skills needed for skin cancer prevention (Guideline 3). Policies that require teaching skin cancer prevention within health education courses will need to be balanced with the overall educational mission of the school.

Policy 6: Policies for Outreach to Families. Schools and other organizations that serve youth have established methods of communicating with parents and other caregivers. Policies can ensure that these organizations routinely provide to their youth advice and information concerning skin cancer prevention. For example, information concerning skin cancer prevention might be distributed along with other health forms to parents at the beginning of the year or at parent and teacher visits.

Policy 7: Resource Allocation and Evaluation. Skin cancer prevention efforts will most likely be sustained if policies exist to guide the allocation of resources for skin cancer prevention. A funding policy usually includes accountability and ongoing evaluation, thus providing for periodic review and reconsideration of how effective the resources dedicated to skin cancer prevention are being used.

Guideline 2: Environmental Change — Provide and Maintain Physical and Social Environments that Support Sun Safety and that are Consistent with the Development of Other Healthful Habits

Policies can promote the provision of supportive resources for skin cancer prevention (e.g., shade, protective clothing and hats, sunscreen at a reduced price or free, and highly visible information and prompts for sun protection) in the physical and social environment. These policies help establish routine personal behaviors and social norms that promote skin cancer prevention in the context of organized group activities.

Physical Environments

The majority of schools in the United States were not designed with sun safety in mind. Sun protection should be considered in the design of new schools. The design of school buildings and adjacent grounds, and the availability of natural shade (e.g., trees and mountains) or constructed shade (e.g., awnings, pavilions, and tall buildings that cast a shadow) influence potential sun exposure. Students, teachers, and families can identify opportunities to extend or create new shaded areas. These areas can be temporary or permanent, natural or constructed. Students might participate in planting trees as part of their science instruction, in which they learn which trees provide good shade cover, how and where to plant them, and how long they will need to yield valuable protection. Existing structures can be modified by constructing roofs on dugouts, installing covers for bleachers, and using awnings and tarps. An increasing selection of portable or add-on shade structures are available that school groups can purchase and install. Major construction projects to build permanent pavilions and play areas can require substantial funding, but they might be the best option in some settings. School and community partnerships can support these endeavors.

School and community partnerships can facilitate provision of sunscreen that is at a reduced price or free for staff and students (through sunscreen manufacturers, pharmaceutical companies, local dermatologist offices, or hospitals) and can make sun safety more accessible during the school day or recreation period. An alternative school policy could encourage parents to apply sunscreen to their children in the morning and include it in their children's supply kits. In addition, schools and community organizations can provide hats and protective clothing (e.g., jackets) for persons who forget to bring their own on days with midday outdoor activity or field trips. Both hygiene, size, and acceptability are important considerations. However, if the school has a laundry facility for band and sports uniforms, a laundering system for emergency sun-safe protective clothing could be instituted.

Information and prompts or reminders can reinforce sun-safety awareness and serve as reminders to engage in skin cancer preventive practices. Both visual and audio messages (e.g., sun-safe posters or public address system announcements) can serve as cues to action for students as well as for families, teachers, and other professionals. After students have learned about the UV index (an indicator of the intensity of the sun's rays on a given day) [124], schools can post and announce the daily UV index to encourage students to practice sun-protection measures. Some schools and recreation settings also use signs that indicate the number of minutes a person can be in the sun before sustaining a sunburn.

Social Environments

A supportive social environment involves establishing social norms favoring skin cancer prevention and including personal preventive behaviors as a part of organized group activities. Program planners and advocates for skin cancer prevention should serve as role models, and adults should be invited to lead by example. Schools can also create a social environment that encourages sun-safety practices through existing peer education groups by having peer educators teach other students about sun safety and by using periodic recognition or a special designation to reward teachers, staff, or students who practice sun safety.

Guideline 3: Education — Provide Health Education to Teach Students the Knowledge, Attitudes, and Behavioral Skills They Need to Prevent Skin Cancer. The Education Should be Age-Appropriate and Linked to Opportunities for Practicing Sun-Safety Behavior

Health education that is designed effectively and implemented for youth can increase their health-related knowledge and contribute to the development of healthy changes in attitudes and behaviors [125]. Skin cancer prevention is likely to be most effective when it is taught as part of a comprehensive health education curriculum that focuses on understanding the relations between personal behavior and health [126] and that provides students with the knowledge and skills outlined by the National Health Education Standards [112].

The yearly timing of skin cancer prevention education can be tailored to the climate and linked with opportunities for sun exposure and sun protection. Therefore, in an area with high altitude where outdoor winter sports are common (e.g., Colorado), skin cancer prevention could be introduced before winter vacation. In northeastern coastal areas, skin cancer prevention might be most relevant before summer break. And during the school day, sun-safety lessons could directly precede recess or outdoor physical education, allowing the class session to be followed by an opportunity to practice positive sun-safety habits.

Skin cancer prevention can be included as part of a comprehensive health education curriculum because of the following characteristics:

- Behaviors that lead to UV radiation exposure might be related to other health risk factors;
- Skin cancer prevention shares many of the key goals of other health education content areas (e.g., increasing the value placed on health, taking responsibility for one's health, and increasing confidence in one's ability to make healthy behavioral changes); and
- Skin cancer prevention efforts can incorporate several of the social learning behavioral change techniques used in other health education domains [126].

In addition to health education classes, skin cancer prevention can be integrated into other subject areas. For example, a math exercise for students could be to calculate the length of safe-sun exposure when sunscreen is used at a certain SPF. In history or social studies classes, students could discuss the social value placed on tanning and fair skin and media portrayal of tanning. Science classes could explore the light spectrum and discuss how it relates to the risk for skin cancer, or discuss depletion of the ozone and its effect on UV exposure. This type of integrated approach requires collaborative planning and curriculum development among teachers to optimize skin cancer prevention education and to ensure consistency of messages and practices.

Scope and Sequence

Health education is most effective in promoting positive behavioral changes when it is repeated and reinforced over time [114]. Short-duration or single-presentation efforts can increase students' knowledge regarding sun safety and, in some cases, improve attitudes and sun-protection behavior immediately after the program. However, these changes are likely to be short-lived and cannot be expected to translate into sustained positive health behaviors [125]. Multiunit presentations have been more effective in achieving higher increases in knowledge and skill acquisition [125].

School-based health education to promote skin cancer prevention is most effective when it is provided consistently and sequentially and included periodically in every grade, from prekindergarten through 12th grade. Sequential instruction can build on information and skills learned previously. Resources for skin cancer prevention programs targeting youth are included in this report (Appendix C).

Active Learning and Behavioral Focus

In the previous decade, educational programs to encourage children to adopt sun-safety habits have been implemented and evaluated. Among the school-based studies reported, interventions have included one-time didactic formats and special events [97,127,128]; skin cancer prevention that is integrated into classroom curricula over time [126,129,130]; and peer-education programs [131,132]. A majority of these studies have demonstrated that these interventions increased knowledge and favorable attitudes toward preventive behaviors. In addition, some of the programs that have multiple lessons and that occur over a longer period (e.g., 1 year) have yielded improvements in sun-protection behaviors [125]

Actively engaging children and adolescents in the learning process increases the likelihood for a positive effect. Youth are more likely to consider and adopt new or improved behaviors when they learn about them through fun, participatory activities rather than through lectures. For example, a recent study demonstrated increased improvement in knowledge of the effects of UV radiation among elementary school students who used an interactive computer-based program than among those who received the same information in a didactic format led by a teacher [133]. The students who completed the interactive CD-ROM program also exhibited significant positive changes in attitudes and a trend toward improvements in sun-safety behavioral scores [133]. The U.S. Environmental Protection Agency offers an Internet learning site where students can report and interpret daily measurements of UV radiation, relate the UV index information to their own community, and correspond with other participating schools [124,134].

Health education activities should be tailored to the cognitive and behavioral level of the students [135]. For example, students in kindergarten through third grades might learn effectively through repetitious rhyming and learning the ABCs of skin cancer prevention. Games, puzzles, and contests make learning fun for students of most ages. More intellectually challenging activities might appeal to high school students, ranging from understanding the scientific basis of solar radiation and global climates, to making their own video to communicate sun-protection messages to their peers and communities. Teenagers can learn about media literacy and different cultures by analyzing images of models in popular magazines and discussing what sun exposure and a tan means to both white and non-white racial groups in the United States and worldwide.

School Programs in a Broader Context

The most important long-term objective of skin cancer prevention education in schools is the adoption and maintenance of sun-protection practices. Therefore, the transmission of detailed, factual information to students is the foundation of sun-safety practices. In addition, educational programs and curricula in schools are part of the broader mix of skin cancer prevention efforts and should not be expected to solely prevent skin cancer. Skin cancer prevention interventions in recreation, sports, and community settings can complement and reinforce efforts in the schools [*120,136–140*]. Supportive policies, environments, teachers, and families are essential adjuncts to effectively planned and consistently implemented health education to prevent skin cancer.

Guideline 4. Family Involvement — Involve Family Members in Skin Cancer Prevention Efforts

The sun-safety practices of parents are the single most important determinant of the sun-protection behaviors of children [121,141]. For younger children, adult family members can assist and provide sun-protection resources. For adolescents, the direct influence of parents might decrease and be subordinated by peer influence. Nonetheless, family support plays a key role in extending the desirable effects of school skin cancer prevention efforts.

Involving family members in skin cancer prevention efforts increases the likelihood that they will adopt and thus model healthful sun-protection behaviors, and also appears to favorably influence the sun-protection behaviors of students [122]. At a minimum, parents or guardians can be informed concerning school initiatives and policies and knowledgeable regarding how their cooperation is needed to ensure child health. Parents and guardians also can be encouraged to provide children with sun-protective clothing and sunglasses for outdoor activities. In addition, parents and guardians can serve as advocates for sun-protective policies and practices in schools and can also provide volunteer labor for health and recreation events. Their input and direct assistance can provide support for funding needed for environmental improvements and educational materials.

Guideline 5: Professional Development — Include Skin Cancer Prevention Knowledge and Skills in Preservice and In-service Education for School Administrators, Teachers, Physical Education Teachers and Coaches, School Nurses, and Others Who Work with Students

Even effectively designed skin cancer prevention programs cannot succeed if they are not implemented as designed. Therefore, appropriate and effective professional development efforts should be conducted for decision makers and caregivers at all levels. Professional development activities, including certification programs and in-service education, are provided routinely for teachers and other school staff (e.g., coaches and school nurses). Skin cancer prevention can be integrated into these activities.

All school staff should receive basic information concerning the importance of sun safety and key strategies for skin cancer prevention. The type of additional professional development needed will vary, depending on the responsibilities of the various caregivers. In-service education for principals might address policy implementation and monitoring, whereas school nurses might highlight proper sunscreen use. Classroom teachers who implement curricula should receive training that addresses both content areas and teaching strategies.

As principals, teachers, and other school staff adopt sun-protection behaviors, they can serve as role models for students. A brief training program, along with participation in conducting skin cancer prevention activities for children, can result in improved sun-protection practices among recreation leaders [142].

Guideline 6: Health Services — Complement and Support Skin Cancer Prevention Education and Sun-Safety Environments and Policies with School Health Services.

School health services provide an opportunity for nurses, health educators, and school health resource specialists to promote and reinforce skin cancer prevention practices. A child's school health record can include parental permission for the child to use sunscreen provided by the school as well as a list of possible allergies to sunscreens or their ingredients.

School health services staff also may conduct physical examinations for sports team eligibility, assist in managing and notifying parents concerning the long-term dangers of a severe sunburn, and prepare students for field trips. Each of these situations provides an opportunity to educate and remind students about skin cancer prevention.

Health professionals in the community, including pediatricians, primary care providers, nurses, pharmacists, and dermatologists are credible sources of information and guidance for skin cancer prevention. They can be advocates for skin cancer prevention policies, environmental changes, and programs, and support school programs through presentations, professional training, demonstrations, and classroom visits. During their consultation with children and parents, these health-care professionals can also assess sun-exposure patterns, reinforce sun-protective behaviors, and provide counseling to persons with sunburns [138,143].

Guideline 7: Evaluation — Periodically Evaluate Whether Schools are Implementing the Guidelines on Policies, Environmental Change, Education, Families, Professional Development, and Health Services

Local school boards and administrators can use evaluation questions to determine whether their programs are consistent with CDC's *Guidelines for School Programs To Prevent Skin Cancer*. Personnel in federal, state, and local education and health agencies also can use these questions to 1) assess whether schools in their jurisdiction are providing effective education to prevent skin cancer and 2) identify schools that would benefit from additional training, resources, or technical assistance. The following questions can serve as a guide for assessing program effectiveness:

1. Do schools have a comprehensive policy on skin cancer prevention and is it implemented and enforced as written?
2. Does the skin cancer prevention program support physical and social environmental changes that promote sun safety and that are consistent with the development of other healthful habits?
3. Does the skin cancer prevention education program foster the necessary knowledge, attitudes, and skills to reduce UV exposure and prevent skin cancer?
4. Is education to reduce UV exposure provided, as planned, in prekindergarten through 12th grade?
5. Is in-service training provided, as planned, for education staff responsible for implementing skin cancer prevention programs?
6. Do school health services support skin cancer prevention?
7. Are parents or families, teachers, students, school health personnel, school administrators, and appropriate community representatives involved in planning, implementing, and assessing programs and policies to prevent skin cancer?
8. Does the skin cancer prevention program encourage and support sun-safety efforts by students and school staff?

CONCLUSION

Schools can play a substantial role in protecting students from unnecessary exposure to UV, thereby reducing their future risk for skin cancer. A comprehensive school approach to skin cancer prevention includes policies, environmental change, educational curricula, family involvement, professional development, integration with health services, and evaluation. The exposure of youth to harmful UV radiation today contributes to their risk for skin cancer later in life. Unlike many diseases, skin cancer is primarily preventable. Schools, in partnership with community groups and other national, federal, state, and voluntary agencies, can develop, implement, and promote initiatives that help protect youth from UV exposure [144,145]. These guidelines serve as a framework for such initiatives.

Appendix A. Public Health Action Steps from the International Agency for Research on Cancer

1. Protection of the skin from solar damage ideally involves various actions that include wearing tightly woven protective clothing that adequately covers the arms, trunk, and legs and a hat that provides adequate shade to the whole of the head; seeking shade whenever possible; avoiding outdoor activities during periods of peak insolation; and using sunscreens. Sunscreens should not be used as the sole agent for protection against the sun.
2. Sunscreens should not be used as a means of extending the duration of solar exposure (e.g., prolonging sunbathing) and it should not be used as a substitute for clothing on sites that are usually unexposed (e.g., the trunk and buttocks).
3. Daily use of sunscreen with a high sun protection factor (>15) on exposed skin is recommended for residents of areas of high insolation who work outdoors or enjoy regular outdoor recreation. Daily use of a sunscreen can reduce the cumulative solar exposure that causes actinic keratoses and squamous cell carcinoma.
4. Adequate solar protection is more important during childhood than any other time in life, and parents and school managers should assiduously apply the first two recommendations.

Source: The International Agency for Research on Cancer Working Group on the Evaluation of Cancer-Preventive Agents. Sunscreens. In: IARC Handbooks of Cancer Prevention. Vol 5. Lyon, France: International Agency for Research on Cancer, 2001.

Appendix B. Sunscreen: How to Select, Apply, and Use It Correctly

When to Apply Sunscreen

- Apply sunscreen approximately 30 minutes before being in the sun (for best results) so that it can be absorbed by the skin and less likely to wash off when you perspire.

- Remember to reapply sunscreen after swimming or strenuous exercise.
- Apply sunscreen often throughout the day if you work outdoors, and wear hats and protective clothing.

How to Apply Sunscreen

- Shake well before use to mix particles that might be clumped up in the container. Consider using the new spray-on or stick types of sunscreen.
- Be sure to apply enough sunscreen. As a rule of thumb, use an ounce (a handful) to cover your entire body.
- Use on all parts of your skin exposed to the sun, including the ears, back, shoulders, and the back of the knees and legs.
- Apply thickly and thoroughly.
- Be careful when applying sunscreen around the eyes.

What to Look for When You Buy Sunscreen

- Pick a broad-spectrum sunscreen that protects against UV-A and UV-B rays and has a sun protection factor (SPF) of at least 15.
- Read product labels. Look for a waterproof brand if you will be sweating or swimming. Buy a nonstinging product or one specifically formulated for your face.
- Buy a brand that does not contain para-aminobenzoic acid (PABA) if you are sensitive to that ingredient.
- Try a sunscreen with different chemicals if your skin reacts badly to the one that you are using. Not all sunscreens have the same ingredients.
- Use a water-based sunscreen if you have oily skin or are prone to acne.
- Be aware that more expensive does not mean better. Although a costly brand might feel or smell better, it is not necessarily more effective than a cheaper product.
- Be aware of the expiration date because some sunscreen ingredients might degrade over time.

APPENDIX C. SKIN CANCER EDUCATION RESOURCES

Skin cancer information and resources are available from various governmental agencies, voluntary organizations, medical associations, and corporations. Information is often available in your state or local area. At the national level, information is available from the sources listed below. The Internet address links take you directly to each organization's skin cancer information section.

American Academy of Dermatology
930 North Meacham Road
P.O. Box 681069
Schaumburg, IL 60173-4965
Phone: 847-330-0230
http://www.aad.org/skincnrUpdates.html

AMC Cancer Research Center
Phone: 800-321-1557
http://www.amc.org/html/market/h_market_sunnydays.html
email: products@amc.org

American Cancer Society
1599 Clifton Road, N.E.
Atlanta, GA 30329
Phone: 800-227-2345
http://www3.cancer.org/cancerinfo

Anti-Cancer Council of Victoria
100 Drummond Street
Carlton Victoria 3053 Australia
Phone: 61-3-9635-5152
Fax: 61-3-9635-5260
http://www.sunsmart.com.au

CDC
National Center for Chronic Disease Prevention and Health Promotion
Division of Cancer Prevention and Control
4770 Buford Highway, N.E.; Mailstop K57

Atlanta, GA 30341-3724
Phone: 770-488-4751
http://www.cdc.gov/cancer/nscpep

National Cancer Institute
Cancer Information Service
Building 31, Room 10A16
31 Center Drive MSC-2580
Bethesda, MD 20892-2580
Phone: 800-422-6237
http://www.cancer.gov

National Council on Skin Cancer Prevention
http://www.skincancerprevention.org

Norris Cotton Cancer Center
The Sun Safe Project
Dartmouth Medical School
Department of Community and Family Medicine
7250 Strasenburgh
Hanover, NH 03755
Phone: 603-650-1566
http://www.dartmouth.edu/dms/sunsafe

U.S. Environmental Protection Agency
Sun Wise School Program
EPA Stratospheric Ozone Information
401 M Street SW (6205J)
Washington, DC 20460
Phone: 800-296-1996
http://www.epa.gov/sunwise

REFERENCES

[1] National Cancer Institute. SEER Cancer Statistics Review, 1973–1998. Available at http://seer.cancer.gov/Publications/CSR1973_1998/melanoma.pdf.

[2] Weinstock, MA; Colditz, GA; Willett, WC; Stampfer, MJ; Bronstein, BR Jr; Speizer, FE. Nonfamilial cutaneous melanoma incidence in women associated with sun exposure before 20 years of age. *Pediatrics*, 1989, 84, 199–204.

[3] Stern, RS; Weinstein, MC,Baker, SG. Risk reduction for nonmelanoma skin cancer with childhood sunscreen use. *Arch Dermatol*, 1986, 122, 537–45.

[4] Gilchrest, BA; Eller, MS; Geller, AC; Yaar, M. The pathogenesis of melanoma induced by ultraviolet radiation. *N Engl J Med*, 1999, 340, 1341–8.

[5] CDC. Guidelines for effective school health education to prevent the spread of AIDS. *MMWR*, 1988, 37(S-2), 1–14.

[6] CDC. Guidelines for school health programs to prevent tobacco use and addiction. *MMWR*, 1994, 43(RR-2), 1–18.

[7] CDC. Guidelines for school health programs to promote lifelong healthy eating. *MMWR*, 1996, 45(RR-9), 1–41.

[8] CDC. Guidelines for school and community programs to promote lifelong physical activity among young people. *MMWR*, 1997, 46(RR-6), 1–36.

[9] CDC. Community guidelines. Available at http://www.thecommunity guide.org/ home_f.html.

[10] US Department of Health and Human Services. Objectives for Improving Health (Part A: Focus Areas 1–14), Cancer. In: Healthy people 2010 (conference ed, Vol 1). Washington, DC: US Department of Health and Human Services 2000, 3-18–3-19. Available at http:// www.health.gov/healthypeople/Document/pdf/Volume1/03Cancer.pdf.

[11] Greenlee, RT; Murray, T; Bolden, S; Wingo, PA. Cancer statistics, 2000. *CA Cancer J Clin*, 2000, 50, 7–33.

[12] American Cancer Society. Cancer prevention and early detection—cancer facts & figures 2002. Atlanta, GA: American Cancer Society, 2002.

[13] Preston, DS; Stern, RS. Nonmelanoma cancers of the skin. *N Engl J Med*, 1992, 327, 1649–62.

[14] Armstrong, BK; English, DR. Cutaneous malignant melanoma. In: Schottenfeld D, Fraumeni JF, eds. Cancer epidemiology and prevention. 2nd ed. New York, NY: Oxford University Press, 1996.

[15] Green, A; MacLennan, R; Youl, P; Martin, N. Site distribution of cutaneous melanoma in Queensland. *Int J Cancer*, 1993, 53, 232–6.

[16] Ries, LA; Wingo, PA; Miller, DS; et al. The annual report to the nation on the status of cancer, 1973–1997, with a special section on colorectal cancer. *Cancer*, 2000, 88, 2398–424.

[17] Jemal, A; Devesa, SS; Hartge, P; Tucker, MA. Recent trends in cutaneous melanoma incidence among whites in the United States. *J Natl Cancer Inst*, 2001, 93, 678-83.

[18] Jemal, A; Devesa, SS; Fears, TR; Hartge, P. Changing patterns of cutaneous malignant melanoma mortality rates among whites in the United States. *J Natl Cancer Inst*, 2000, 92, 811–8.

[19] Hall, HI; Miller, DR; Rogers, JD; Bewerse, B. Update on the incidence and mortality from melanoma in the United States. *J Am Acad Dermatol*, 1999, 40, 35–42. Available at http://seer.cancer.gov/Publications/CSR1973_1998/melanoma.pdf.

[20] Armstrong, BK; Kricker, A. How much melanoma is caused by sun exposure?. *Melanoma Res*, 1993, 3, 395–401.

[21] Diffey, BL. Solar ultraviolet radiation effects on biological systems. *Phys Med Biol*, 1991, 36, 299–328.

[22] IARC Working Group on the Evaluation of Cancer-Preventive Agents. Sunscreens. In: IARC Handbooks of Cancer Prevention. Vol 5. Lyon, France: International Agency for Research on Cancer, 2001.

[23] Taylor, HR; West, SK; Rosenthal, FS; et al. Effect of ultraviolet radiation on cataract formation. *N Engl J Med*, 1988, 319, 1429–33.

[24] West, SK; Duncan, DD; Munoz, B, et al. Sunlight exposure and risk of lens opacities in a population-based study: the Salisbury Eye Evaluation project. *JAMA*, 1998, 280, 714–8.

[25] Rosmini, F; Stazi, MA; Milton, Rc; Sperduto, RD; Pasquini, P; Maraini, G. A dose-response effect between a sunlight index and age-related cataracts. Italian-American Cataract Study Group. *Ann Epidemiol*, 1994, 4, 266–70.

[26] Whiteman, DC; Whiteman, CA; Green, AC. Childhood sun exposure as a risk factor for melanoma: a systematic review of epidemiologic studies. *Cancer Causes Control*, 2001, 12, 69–82.

[27] Westerdahl, J; Olsson, H; Ingvar, C. At what age do sunburn episodes play a crucial role for the development of malignant melanoma. *Eur J Cancer*, 1994, 30A, 1647–54.

[28] Elwood, JM; Jopson, J. Melanoma and sun exposure: an overview of published studies. *Int J Cancer*, 1997, 73, 198–203.

[29] Kricker, A; Armstrong, BK; English, DR. Sun exposure and non-melanocytic skin cancer. *Cancer Causes Control*, 1994, 5, 367–92.

[30] Kricker, A; Armstrong, BK; English, DR; Heenan, PJ. Does intermittent sun exposure cause basal cell carcinoma? A case-control study in Western Australia. *Int J Cancer*, 1995, 60, 489–94.

[31] Gallagher, RP; Hill, GB; Bajdik, CD; et al. Sunlight exposure, pigmentary factors, and risk of nonmelanocytic skin cancer I. Basal cell carcinoma. *Arch Dermatol*, 1995, 131, 157–63.

[32] Gallagher RP. Sun exposure and non-melanocytic skin cancer. In: Grob JJ, Stern RS, MacKie RM, Weinstock WA, eds. Epidemiology, causes and prevention of skin diseases. 1st ed. London, England: Blackwell Science, 1997, 72–7.

[33] Armstrong, BK. Melanoma: childhood or lifelong sun exposure. In: Grob JJ, Stern RS, Mackie RM, Weinstock WA, eds. Epidemiology, causes and prevention of skin diseases. 1st ed. London, England: Blackwell Science, 1997, 63–6.

[34] Whiteman, D; Green, A. Melanoma and sunburn. *Cancer Causes Control*, 1994, 5, 564–72.

[35] Autier, P; Dore, JF; Cattaruzza, MS; et al. Sunscreen use, wearing clothes, and number of nevi in 6to 7-year-old European children. European Organization for Research and Treatment of Cancer Melanoma Cooperative Group. *J Nat Cancer Inst*, 1998, 90, 1873–80.

[36] Buller, DB; Callister, MA; Reichert, T. Skin cancer prevention by parents of young children: health information sources, skin cancer knowledge, and sun-protection practices. *Oncol Nurs Forum*, 1995, 22, 1559–66.

[37] Foltz, AT. Parental knowledge and practices of skin cancer prevention: a pilot study. *J Pediatr Health Care*, 1993, 7, 220–5.

[38] Hurwitz, S. The sun and sunscreen protection: recommendations for children. *J Dermatol Surg Oncol*, 1988, 14, 657–60.

[39] Taylor, CR; Stern, RS; Leyden, JJ; Gilchrest, BA. Photoaging/ photodamage and photoprotection. *J Am Acad Dermatol*, 1990, 22, 1–15.

[40] Autier, P; Dore, JF. Influence of sun exposures during childhood and during adulthood on melanoma risk. EPIMEL and EORTC Melanoma Cooperative Group. European Organization for Research and Treatment of Cancer. *Int J Cancer.*, 1998, 77, 533–7.

[41] Williams, ML; Pennella, R. Melanoma, melanocytic nevi, and other melanoma risk factors in children. *J Pediatr*, 1994, 124, 833–45.

[42] Parkin, DM; Muir, CS; Whelan, SL; Gao, YT; Ferlay, J; Powell, J. *Cancer incidence in five continents*. Vol 6. Lyon, France: International Agency for Research on Cancer, 1992.

[43] Scotto, J; Fears, TR; Freaumeni, JF, Jr. Incidence of nonmelanoma skin cancer in the United States. Washington, DC: US Department of Health and Human Services, Public Health Service, National Institutes of Health, National Cancer Institute, 1981: DHHS publication no. (NIH) 83-2433.

[44] Pennello, G; Devesa, S; Gail, M. Association of surface ultraviolet B radiation levels with melanoma and nonmelanoma skin cancer in United States blacks. *Cancer Epidemiol Biomarkers Prev*, 2000, 9, 291–7.

[45] Rhodes, AR; Weinstock, MA; Fitzpatrick, TB; Mihm, MC, Jr; Sober, AJ. Risk factors for cutaneous melanoma. A practical method of recognizing predisposed individuals. *JAMA*, 1987, 258, 3146–54.

[46] Scotto, J; Fears, TR; Kraemer, KH; Fraumeni, JF. Nonmelanoma skin cancer. In: Schottenfeld D, Fraumeni JF, eds. Cancer epidemiology and prevention. 2nd ed. New York, NY: Oxford University Press, 1996.

[47] Kricker, A; Armstrong, BK; English, DR; Heenan, PJ. Pigmentary and cutaneous risk factors for non-melanocytic skin cancer—a case-control study. *Int J Cancer*, 1991, 48, 650–62.

[48] Holly, EA; Kelly, JW; Shpall, SN; Chiu, SH. Number of melanocytic nevi as a major risk factor for malignant melanoma. *J Am Acad Dermatol*, 1987, 17, 459–68.

[49] Holly, EA; Kelly, JW; Ahn, DK; Shpall, SV; Rosen, JI. Risk of cutaneous melanoma by number of melanocytic nevi and correlation of nevi by anatomic site. In: Gallagher RP, Elwood JM, eds. Epidemiological aspects of cutaneous malignant melanoma. Boston, MA: Kluwer Academic Publishers, 1994, 159–72.

[50] Goldstein, AM; Tucker, MA. Genetic epidemiology of familial melanoma. *Dermatol Clin*, 1995, 35, 605–12.

[51] National Cancer Institute. *Canques*. Available at http://seer.cancer.gov/ScientificSystems/CanQues.

[52] International Agency for Research on Cancer. Solar and ultraviolet radiation. *IARC Monogr Eval Carcinog Risks Hum*, 1992, 55, 1–316.

[53] Koh, HK; Sinks, TH; Geller, AC; Miller, DR; Lew, RA. Etiology of melanoma. In: Nathanson L, ed. *Current research and clinical management of melanoma*. Boston, MA: Kluwer Academic Publishers, 1993, 1–27.

[54] Diffey, BL. Ozone Depletion and skin cancer. In: Grob JJ, Stern RS, Mackie RM, Weinstock WA, eds. Epidemiology, causes and prevention of skin diseases. 1st ed. London, England: Blackwell Science, 1997, 77–85.
[55] National Institute of Environmental Health Sciences. Report on carcinogens: solar UV radiation and exposure to sunbeds and sunlamps. 9th ed. Research Triangle Park, NC, 2000, 48–50.
[56] Swerdlow, AJ; Weinstock, MA. Do tanning lamps cause melanoma? An epidemiologic assessment. *J Am Acad Dermatol*, 1998, 38, 89–98.
[57] Miller, SA; Hamilton, SL; Wester, UG; Cyr, WH. An analysis of UVA emissions from sunlamps and the potential importance for melanoma. *Photochem Photobiol*, 1998, 68, 63–70.
[58] Spencer, JM; Amonette, RA. Indoor tanning: risks, benefits, and future trends. *J Am Acad Dermatol*, 1995, 33, 288–98.
[59] Saraiya, M; Frank, E; Elon, L; Baldwin, G; McAlpine, BE. Personal and clinical skin cancer prevention practices of U.S. women physicians. *Arch Derm*, 2000, 136, 633–42.
[60] McDonald, CJ. American Cancer Society perspective on the American College of Preventive Medicine's policy statements on skin cancer prevention and screening. *CA Cancer J Clin*, 1998, 48, 229–31.
[61] Committee on Guidelines of Care, American Academy of Dermatology. Guidelines of care for cutaneous squamous cell carcinoma. *J Am Acad Dermatol*, 1993, 28, 628–31.
[62] Committee on Guidelines of Care, American Academy of Dermatology. Guidelines of care for nevi I (nevocellular nevi and seborrheic keratoses). *J Am Acad Dermatol*, 1992, 26, 629–31.
[63] Committee on Environmental Health, American Academy of *Pediatrics*. Ultraviolet light: a hazard to children. *Pediatrics*, 1999, 104, 328–33.
[64] Council on Scientific Affairs. Harmful effects of ultraviolet radiation. *JAMA*, 1989, 262, 380–4.
[65] National Cancer Institute. Skin cancer (PDQ®): Prevention. Available at http://www.cancer.gov/cancer_information/doc_pdq.aspx?version=patient&viewid=dd7fa1a5-9c70-4625-9112-d2db13af013d.
[66] Autier, P; Dore, JF; Shifflers, E; et al. Melanoma and use of sunscreens: an EORTC case-control study in Germany, Belgium, and France. The EORTC Melanoma Cooperative Group. *Int J Cancer*, 1995, 61, 749–55.
[67] Welsh, C; Diffey, BL. The protection against solar actinic radiation afforded by common clothing fabrics. *Clinical Exp Dermatol*, 1981, 6, 577–82.

[68] Pailthorpe, M. Apparel textiles and sun protection: a marketing opportunity or a quality control nightmare? *Mutat Res*, 1998, 422, 175–83.

[69] Diffey, BL; Cheeseman, J. Sun protection with hats. *Br J Dermatol*, 1992, 127, 10–12.

[70] American Sun Protection Organization. Sun safety info: clothing. Available at http://www.americansun.org/pages/clothing.htm.

[71] Gies, HP; Roy, CR; Elliott, G; Zongli, W. Ultraviolet radiation protection factors for clothing. *Health Phys*, 1994, 67, 131–9.

[72] American Academy of Ophthalmology. Sunglasses. San Francisco, CA: American Academy of Ophthalmology, 1995.

[73] Gies, HP; Roy, CR; Elliot, G. Ultraviolet radiation protection factors for personal protection in both occupational and recreational situations. *Radiat Prot Aust*, 1992, 10, 59–66.

[74] Greenwood, JS; Soulos, GP; Thomas, ND. Under cover: guidelines for shade planning and design. Sydney, Australia: New South Wales Cancer Council and New South Wales Health Department, 1998.

[75] Parsons, PG; Neale, R; Wolski, P; Green, A. The shady side of solar protection. *Med J Aust*, 1998, 168, 327–30.

[76] Vainio, H; Miller, AB; Bianchini, F. An international evaluation of the cancer-preventive potential of sunscreens. *Int J Cancer*, 2000, 88, 838–42.

[77] Thompson, SC; Jolley, D; Marks, R. Reduction of solar keratoses by regular sunscreen use. *N Engl J Med*, 1993, 329, 1147–51.

[78] Naylor, MF; Boyd, A; Smith, DW; Cameron, GS; Hubbard, D; Neldner, KH. High sun protection factor sunscreens in the suppression of actinic neoplasia. *Arch Dermatol*, 1995, 131, 170–5.

[79] Green, A; Williams, G; Neale, R; et al. Daily sunscreen application and betacarotene supplementation in prevention of basal-cell and squamous-cell carcinomas of the skin: a randomised controlled trial. *Lancet*, 1999, 354, 723–9.

[80] Gallagher, RP; Rivers, JK; Lee, TK; Bajdik, CD; McLean, DI; Coldman, AJ. Broad-spectrum sunscreen use and the development of new nevi in white children: a randomized controlled trial. *JAMA*, 2000, 283, 2955–60.

[81] Weinstock, MA. Do sunscreens increase or decrease melanoma risk: an epidemiologic evaluation. *J Invest Dermatol Symp Proc*, 1999, 4, 97–100.

[82] McLean, DI; Gallagher, R. Sunscreens: use and misuse. *Dermatol Clin*, 1998, 16, 219–26.

[83] Odio, MR; Veres, DA; Goodman, JJ; et al. Comparative efficacy of sunscreen reapplication regimens in children exposed to ambient sunlight. *Photodermatol Photoimmunol Photomed*, 1994, 10, 118–25.

[84] Baade, PD; Balanda, KP; Lowe, JB. Changes in skin protection behaviors, attitudes, and sunburn: in a population with the highest incidence of skin cancer in the world. *Cancer Detect Prev*, 1996, 20, 566–75.

[85] Bech-Thomsen, N; Wulf, HC. Sunbathers' application of sunscreen is probably inadequate to obtain the sun protection factor assigned to the preparation. *Photodermatol Photoimmunol Photomed*, 1992–1993, 9, 242–44.

[86] Sayre, RM; Kollias, N; Ley, RD; Baqer, AH. Changing the risk spectrum of injury and the performance of sunscreen products throughout the day. *Photodermatol Photoimmnol Photomed*, 1994, 10, 148–53.

[87] Foley, P; Nixon, R; Marks, R; Frower, K; Thompson, S. The frequency of reactions to sunscreens: results of a longitudinal population-based study on the regular use of sunscreens in Australia. *Br J Dermatol*, 1993, 128, 512–8.

[88] Keesling, B,Friedman, HS. Psychosocial factors in sunbathing and sunscreen use. *Health Psychol*, 1987, 6, 477–93.

[89] Randle, HW. Suntanning: differences in perceptions throughout history. *Mayo Clinic Proc*, 1997, 72, 461–6.

[90] Chapman, S; Marks, R; King, M. Trends in tans and skin protection in Australian fashion magazines 1982 through 1991. *Am J Public Health*, 1992, 82, 1677–80.

[91] Johnson, EY; Lookingbill, DP. Sunscreen use and sun exposure: trends in a white population. *Arch Dermatol*, 1984, 120, 727–31.

[92] Banks, BA; Silverman, RA; Schwartz, RH; Tunnessen, WW, Jr. Attitudes of teenagers toward sun exposure and sunscreen use. *Pediatrics*, 1992, 89, 40–2.

[93] Lescano, CM; Rodrique, JR. Skin cancer prevention behaviors among parents of young children. *Children's Health Care*, 1997, 26, 107–14.

[94] Hall, HI; May, DS; Lew, RA; Koh, HK; Nadel, M. Sun protection behaviors of the U.S. white population. *Prev Med*, 1997, 26, 401–7.

[95] Hall, HI; Rogers, JD. Sun protection behaviors among African Americans. *Ethn Dis*, 1999, 9, 126–31.

[96] Marks, R. Role of childhood in the development of skin cancer. *Aust Paediatr J*, 1988, 24, 337–8.

[97] Mermelstein, RJ; Riesenberg, LA. Changing knowledge and attitudes about skin cancer risk factors in adolescents. *Health Psychol*, 1992, 11, 371–6.

[98] Reynolds, KD; Blaum, JM; Jester, PM; Weiss, H; Soong, SJ; Diclemente, RJ. Predictors of sun exposure in adolescents in southeastern U.S. population. *J Adolesc Health*, 1996, 19, 409–15.

[99] Robinson, JK; Rigel, DS; Amonette, RA. Trends in sun exposure knowledge, attitudes, and behaviors: 1986 to 1996. *J Am Acad Dermatol*, 1997, 37, 179–86.

[100] Jorgensen, CM; Wayman, J; Green, C; Gelb, CA. Using health communications for primary prevention of skin cancer: CDC's Choose Your Cover campaign. *J Womens Health Gend Based Med*, 2000, 9, 471–5.

[101] Hall, HI; Jones, SE; Saraiya, M. Prevalence and correlates of sunscreen use among US high school students. *J Sch Health*, 2001, 71, 453–7.

[102] Glanz, K; Lew, R; Song, V; Ah, Cook, VA. Factors associated with skin cancer prevention practices in a multiethnic population. *Health Educ Behav*, 1999, 26, 344–59.

[103] Maducdoc, LR; Wagner, RF, Jr; Wagner, KD. Parents' use of sunscreen on beach-going children: the burnt child dreads the fire. *Arch Dermatol*, 1982, 128, 628–9.

[104] Grob, JJ; Guglielmina, C; Gouvernet, J; Zarour, H; Noe, C; Bonerandi, JJ. Study of sunbathing habits in children and adolescents: application to the prevention of melanoma. *Dermatology*, 1993, 186, 94–8.

[105] Vail-Smith, K; Watson, CL; Felts, WM; Parrillo, AV; Knight, SM; Hughes JL. Childhood sun exposure: parental knowledge, attitudes, and behaviors. *J Health Educ*, 1997, 28, 149–55.

[106] Olson, AL; Dietrich, AJ; Sox, CH; Stevens, MM; Winchell, CW; Ahles, TA. Solar protection of children at the beach. *Pediatrics*, 1997, 99, E1.

[107] Hall, HI; McDavid, K; Jorgensen, CM; Kraft, JM. Factors associated with sunburn in white children aged 6 months to 11 years. Am J *Prev Med*, 2001, 20, 9–14.

[108] Robinson, JK; Rigel, DS; Amonette, RA. Summertime sun protection used by adults for their children. *J Am Acad Dermatol*, 2000, 42, 746–53.

[109] Standing Committee on the Scientific Evaluation of Dietary Reference Intakes, Institute of Medicine. Dietary reference intakes for calcium, phosphorus, magnesium, vitamin D, and fluoride. Washington, DC: National Academy Press, 1997.

[110] Vieth, R. Vitamin D supplementation, 25-hydroxyvitamin D concentrations and safety. *Am J Clin Nutr*, 1999, 69, 842–56.

[111] American Academy of Pediatrics. Vitamins: vitamin D. In: Kleinman RE, ed. Pediatric nutrition handbook, 4th ed. Elk Grove Village, IL: American Academy of Pediatrics, 1998, 275–7.

[112] Joint Committee on National Health Education Standards. National health education standards: achieving health literacy—an investment in the future. Atlanta, GA: American Cancer Society, 1995.

[113] McKenzie, FD; Richmond, JB. Linking health and learning: an overview of coordinated school health programs. In: Marx E, Wooley SF, eds. Health is academic: a guide to coordinated school health programs. New York, NY: Teachers College Press, 1998.

[114] Carlyon, P; Carlyon, W; McCarthy, AR. Family and community involvement in school health. In: Marx E, Wooley SF, eds. Health is academic: a guide to coordinated school health programs. New York, NY: Teachers College Press, 1998.

[115] Glanz, K; Lewis, FM; Rimer, BK; eds. Health behavior and health education: theory, research and practice. 2nd ed. San Francisco, CA: JosseyBass Inc, 1997.

[116] Henderson, A; Rowe, DE. *A healthy school environment*. In: Marx E, Wooley SF, eds. Health is academic: a guide to coordinated school health programs. New York, NY: Teachers College Press, 1998.

[117] Glanz, K; Lankenau, B; Foerster, S; Temple, S; Mullis, R; Schmid, T. Environmental and policy approaches to cardiovascular disease prevention through nutrition: opportunities for state and local action. *Health Educ Qtly*, 1995, 22, 512–27.

[118] Sallis, JF; Owen, N. Ecological models. In: Glanz K, Lewis FM, Rimer BK, eds. Health behavior and health education: theory, research and practice. 2nd ed. San Francisco, CA: Jossey-Bass Inc, 1997, 403–24.

[119] Queensland, Cancer, Fund. Working towards a SunSmart Queensland. Queensland, Australia: Queensland Cancer Fund, 1997.

[120] Schofield, MJ; Edwards, K; Pearce, R. Effectiveness of two strategies for dissemination of sun-protection policy in New South Wales primary and secondary schools. *Aust N Z J Public Health*, 1997, 21, 743–50.

[121] Glanz, K; Carbone, E; Song, V. Formative research for developing targeted skin cancer prevention programs for children in multiethnic Hawaii. *Health Education Research*, 1999, 14, 155–66.

[122] Glanz, K; Lew, RA; Song, V; Murakami-Akatsuka, L. Skin cancer prevention program in outdoor recreation settings: effects of the Hawaii SunSmart Program. *Effective Clinical Practice*, 2000, 3, 53–61.

[123] Wolf, SM; Swanson, LA; Manning, R. PROJECT SPF (Sun Safety, Protection and Fun): Arizona Department of Health Services Early Childhood Skin Cancer Prevention Education Program. *Health Educ Behav*, 1999, 26, 301–5.

[124] United States Environmental Protection Agency. The SunWise School Program Guide. Available at http://www.epa.gov/sunwise/guide.pdf.

[125] Buller, DB; Borland, R. Skin cancer prevention for children: a critical review. *Health Educ Behav*, 1999, 26, 317–43.

[126] Buller, MK; Loescher, LJ; Buller, DB. Sunshine and Skin Health: a curriculum for skin cancer prevention education. *J Cancer Educ*, 1994, 9, 155–62.

[127] Buller, MK; Goldberg, G; Buller, DB. Sun Smart Day: a pilot program for photoprotection education. Pediatric Dermatol, 1997, 14, 257–63.

[128] Thornton, CM; Piacquadio, DJ. Promoting sun awareness: evaluation of an educational children's book. *Pediatrics*, 1996, 98, 52–5.

[129] Buller, DB; Buller, MK; Beach, B; Ertl, G. Sunny days, healthy ways: evaluation of a skin cancer prevention curriculum for elementary schoolaged children. *J Am Acad Dermatol*, 1996, 35, 911–22.

[130] Girgis, A; Sanson-Fisher, RW; Tripodi, DA; Golding, T. Evaluation of interventions to improve solar protection in primary schools. *Health Educ Qtly*, 1993, 20, 275–87.

[131] Fork, HE; Wagner, RF; Wagner, KD. The Texas peer education sun awareness project for children: primary prevention of malignant melanoma and nonmelanocytic skin cancers. *Cutis*, 1992, 50, 363–4.

[132] Reding, DJ; Fischer, V; Gunderson, P; Lappe, K. Skin cancer prevention: a peer education model. *Wisc Med J*, 1995, 94, 75–9.

[133] Hornung, RL; Lennon, PA; Garrett, JM; DeVellis, RF; Weinberg PD, Strecher, VJ. Interactive computer technology for skin cancer prevention targeting children. *Amer J Prev Med*, 2000, 18, 69–76.

[134] Cantor, MA; Rosseel, K. The United States Environmental Protection Agency SunWise School Program. *Health Educ Behav*, 1999, 26, 303–4.

[135] Perry, CL. Creating health behavior change: how to develop community-wide programs for youth. *Thousand Oaks*, CA: Sage, 1999.

[136] Mayer, JA; Slymen, DJ; Eckhardt, L; et al. Reducing ultraviolet radiation exposure in children. *Prev Med*, 1997, 26, 516–22.
[137] Parrott, R; Duggan, A; Cremo, J; Eckles, A; Jones, K; Steiner, C. Communicating about youth's sun exposure risk to soccer coaches and parents: a pilot study in Georgia. *Health Educ Behav*, 1999, 26, 385–95.
[138] Dietrich, AJ; Olson, AL; Sox, CH; et al. A community-based randomized trial encouraging sun protection for children. *Pediatrics*, 1998, 102, E64.
[139] Dietrich, AJ; Olson, AL; Sox, CH; Tosteson, TD; Grant-Petersson, J. Persistent increase in children's sun protection in a randomized controlled community trial. *Prev Med*, 2000, 31, 569–74.
[140] Miller, DR; Geller, AC; Wood, MC; Lew, RA; Koh, HK. The Falmouth Safe Skin Project: evaluation of a community program to promote sun protection in youth. *Health Educ Behav*, 1999, 26, 369–84.
[141] Arthey, S; Clarke, VA. Suntanning and sun protection: a review of the psychological literature. *Soc Sci Med*, 1995, 40, 265–74.
[142] Glanz, K; Maddock, J; Lew, RA; Murakami-Akatsuka, L. A randomized trial of the Hawaii SunSmart program's impact on outdoor recreation staff. *J Am Acad Dermatol*, 2001, 44, 973–8.
[143] Easton, AN; Price, JH; Boehm, K; Telljohann, SK. Sun protection counseling by pediatricians. *Arch Pediatr Adolesc Med*, 1997, 151, 1133–8.
[144] Green, LW; Kreuter, MW. Health promotion planning: an educational and ecological approach. 3rd ed. Mountain View, CA: Mayfield Publishing, 1999.
[145] Hill, D; Dixon, H. Promoting sun protection in children: rationale and challenges. *Health Educ Behav*, 1999, 26, 409–17.

In: Sun Safety for Schools and Youth
Editor: Jarrod C. Walton

ISBN: 978-1-63463-067-2

Chapter 2

SHADE PLANNING FOR AMERICA'S SCHOOLS[*]

Centers for Disease Control and Prevention

WHAT IS THE PURPOSE OF THIS MANUAL?

In 2002, the Centers for Disease Control and Prevention (CDC) published the *Guidelines for School Programs to Prevent Skin Cancer*, which outlines steps that school communities can take to develop a comprehensive approach to reducing the risk for skin cancer among students, teachers, staff, and visitors. The guidelines include the following recommendations:

- Establish policies that reduce exposure to solar ultraviolet (UV) radiation.
- Provide and maintain physical and social environments that support sun safety.
- Provide opportunities for students to gain the knowledge, develop the attitudes, and practice the skills needed to prevent skin cancer.
- Involve family members in skin cancer prevention efforts.

[*] This is an edited, reformatted and augmented version of a report prepared under contract for the Centers for Disease Control and Prevention, National Center for Chronic Disease Prevention and Health, Division of Cancer Prevention and Control, 2008.

- Provide pre-service and in-service skin cancer prevention education for school administrators, teachers, coaches, school nurses, and other professionals who work with students.
- Support sun-safety policies, sun-safe environments, and skin cancer prevention education with school health services.
- Evaluate the implementation of policies, environmental change, education, family involvement, professional development, and health services.

This manual has been created to support school communities in their implementation of the *Guidelines for School Programs to Prevent Skin Cancer* and, specifically, to help schools create and maintain a physical environment that supports sun safety by ensuring that school grounds have adequate shade.

Between 68% and 90% of all melanomas result from exposure to ultraviolet radiation.[1]

Why Should Schools Care About Skin Cancer?

Cancer of the skin is the most commonly diagnosed cancer in the United States and perhaps the most preventable. Melanoma and non-melanoma cancers, including basal cell cancer and squamous cell cancer, account for as much as 50% of all cancers. Because the reporting of non-melanoma cancers to cancer registries is not required, the exact number of non-melanoma cancer cases is not known. However, estimates indicate that as many as 1 million cases of basal cell and squamous cell skin cancer occur each year.[2] Melanoma, which accounts for only about 5% of skin cancer cases, also accounts for 79% of skin cancer deaths. From 1973 and through the early eighties, the incidence rate of melanoma among white men and women in the United States increased by about 6% per year. Since the early eighties, the increase has been around 3% annually. Approximately 55,100 new melanomas were diagnosed in the United States in 2004, and about 7,910 people died of melanoma that same year.[3]

Almost all of these cancers are preventable.[4] In most cases, exposure to solar UV radiation is the cause of the cancer. Using multiple methods for estimating the incidence of melanoma that might be attributable to exposure to the sun, Armstrong and Kricker, reporting in *Melanoma Research*, suggest that between 68% and 90% of all melanomas result from exposure to UV radiation.[5]

> **SOLAR RADIATION ADDED TO THE LIST OF "KNOWN" CARCINOGENS**
>
> The federal government's 11th edition of the Report on Carcinogens listed the sun and any other source of broad spectrum ultraviolet radiation as "known" causes of cancer.
>
> "The report cites data indicating a cause-and-effect relationship between this radiation and skin cancer, cancer of the lip and melanoma of the eye. The report goes on to say that skin cancers are observed with increasing duration of exposure and for those who experience sunburn."
>
> From National Institutes of Health News Release dated December 11, 2002

Why Shade?

There are many reasons that a school might want to improve the quality and increase the amount of accessible shade on school grounds. The most obvious and one of the most important reasons is that shade provides protection from solar UV radiation. Due to the scheduling complexities of physical education classes, sporting events, and other outdoor activities, students are often exposed to solar UV radiation during the peak sun hours of the day—between 10:00 a.m. and 4:00 p.m. For some schools and for some students, using sun protective methods, such as hats or sunscreen, or implementing policy changes could prove to be problematic. Providing shade in areas where students already participate in outdoor activities can afford passive protection from the sun's damaging rays.

What Are the Additional Benefits of Shade?

Extending the Classroom

Schools are often looking for ways to extend their classrooms. Two strategies for increasing shade on school grounds can also help schools create novel classroom experiences for their students. These strategies may be employed independently or in concert. The first is to modify existing structures or build new ones to provide shade where students play and socialize. The second calls for the strategic planting of additional shade-producing trees, vines, and shrubs. Structures built to provide shade can also be designed as covered outdoor learning areas, thereby extending the classroom beyond the school walls. Planting shade-producing vegetation affords schools the opportunity to create and maintain natural outdoor classrooms where students can enjoy hands-on experiences in the natural world. Both strategies could potentially provide teachers with new ideas for curricula and new reasons to take their students outdoors.

Extended Periods of Physical Activity

In adults, regular physical activity is linked to enhanced health and reduced risk for the development of many chronic diseases. Lifelong physical activity patterns are often developed in childhood and adolescence. In the section on preventing physical activity-related injuries in *CDC's Guidelines for School and Community Programs to Promote Lifelong Physical Activity Among Young People,* the use of shaded spaces or indoor facilities to reduce the incidence of heat-related illnesses is recommended. Not all schools have indoor facilities designed for active play; however, providing shade on existing outdoor play areas could reduce the temperature in those areas by as much as 10° to 20 °, increasing the period of time that students could engage in active outdoor play.

School Grounds Aesthetics

All too often, school grounds are an environment of concrete, asphalt, steel, turf grass, and chain link fences. In planning strategies to provide or increase shade on school grounds, schools have a second chance to improve the aesthetics of the school property, making the grounds more inviting to students, teachers, staff, parents, and visitors. A well-planned shade implementation project engages the entire school community in making the school a more pleasant place to learn.

Who Should Read This Manual?

A school includes not just the principal, teachers, students, and staff, but also key stakeholders and decision-makers that comprise the school community. In addition to school officials, the school community includes parents, neighbors, and members of the broader community, all of whom have a stake in helping to protect the community's children and adolescents from skin cancer. This manual was written as a reference tool for the entire school community, encompassing both the school district and the individual school.

How Can This Manual Be Used?

Section 1 School board members, superintendents, principals, and school health advisory councils can use this manual to acquaint themselves with issues relating to the damaging effects of solar UV radiation, skin cancer prevention, and planning for shade implementation at their schools. The first section gives information on both the short- and long-term effects of UV radiation on health and provides a rationale for developing sun-safe policies in schools.

Section 2 The second section addresses strategies for providing shade at schools and includes some of the advantages and disadvantages of each strategy. School board members, superintendents, principals, school health advisory councils, and school shade planning teams will find this information useful in determining the strategies that will work best at their school.

Section 3 The third section presents an overview of the process of planning a shade implementation project. School board members, superintendents, principals, and school health advisory councils can use it as a brief overview of the process. School shade planning teams can refer to this section for an introduction to the process and to sections 4 and 6 for more detailed information to guide them through the steps of shade planning.

Section 4 The fourth section presents information about schools and school districts that have engaged in shade planning projects and reveals some successful strategies. The needs of every school differ; there is no one-size-fits-all solution to providing shade at schools. This section offers a glimpse of shade strategies that others have employed.

Section 5 The fifth section gives the reader a basic introduction, or reintroduction, to solar geometry and the relationship between the Earth and Sun. Illustrations are included showing the effects of daily and seasonal changes in solar angles on the length and direction of shadows.

Section 6 The sixth section guides shade planning team members through the process of conducting a shade audit. The shade audit allows planning teams to consider the needs of the school in relation to the quantity and quality of shade already available to students, teachers, and staff.

SECTION 1. WHAT IS UV RADIATION?

Ultraviolet (UV) radiation is one component of a broad spectrum of electromagnetic radiation emitted by the sun. The spectrum also includes visible light, which we see, and infrared radiation, which we feel as heat.

The ultraviolet area of the spectrum can be further divided into three bands, ultraviolet A (UVA), ultraviolet B (UVB), and ultraviolet C (UVC). All UVC radiation and almost all UVB radiation are absorbed in the ozone layer of the atmosphere. UVA radiation penetrates the atmosphere unimpeded and, until recently, had been considered innocuous.

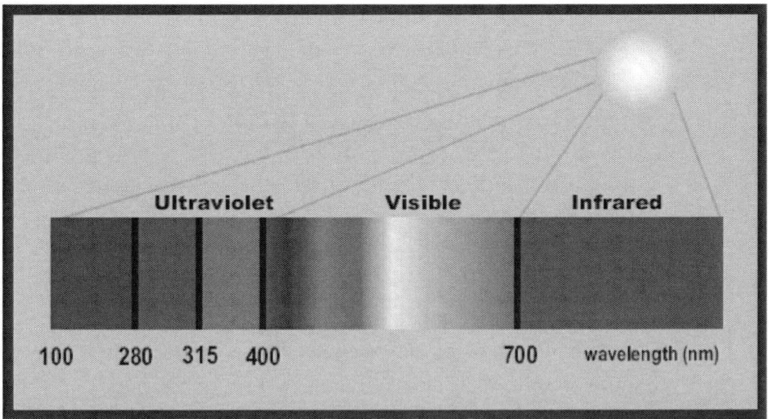

The Sun's Radiation Spectrum

What Are the Factors That Affect UV Radiation Levels?

Time of Day

At solar noon, the sun is at its highest point of the day. As much as 30% of total UV radiation is received in the hour before and the hour after solar noon, and as much as 75% is received during the 3 hours before and the 3 hours after solar noon.[6]

Time of Year

Because the angles of the sun change throughout the year, the intensity of UV radiation changes as well. In the northern hemisphere, UV radiation tends to be greater in the summer months.

SHADE PLANNING TOOLBOX

Q: What time is solar noon?

A: That depends on the day of the year, your latitude and longitude, and your location within your time zone.

On July 4, solar noon is at:
- 12:48 (EDT) in Boston
- 1:40 (EDT) in Knoxville
- 12:51 (CDT) in Nashville
- 12:53 (PDT) in San Diego

On February 1, solar noon is at:
- 11:57 (EST) in Boston
- 12:49 (EST) in Knoxville
- 12:00 (CST) in Nashville
- 12:02 (PST) in San Diego

To find out what time solar noon occurs on any day of the year at any location, visit the National Oceanic and Atmospheric Administration (NOAA) Surface Radiation Research Branch web site at http://www.srrb.noaa.gov/ highlights/sunrise/sunrise.html.

Geographical Latitude

UV radiation decreases as the distance from the equator increases.

Altitude

Because the atmosphere is thinner at higher altitudes and less able to absorb UVB, total UV radiation is greater at higher altitudes.

Weather Conditions

Although clouds reduce the full spectrum of solar radiation, they do not reduce UV radiation to the same extent that they reduce visible light and infrared radiation. Clouds may make us feel cooler and block our view of the sun, but they do not fully protect us from UV radiation.

Atmospheric Ozone

The stratosphere's ozone layer provides us with an enormous amount of protection against the damaging effects of UV radiation. Unfortunately, in certain areas, ozone has been depleted to a dangerous extent, primarily due to the release of chlorofluorocarbons (CFCs) and other ozone-depleting chemicals, such as carbon tetrachloride and methyl chloroform, into the atmosphere. Both carbon tetrachloride and methyl chloroform are solvents that have been used in industrial applications, and CFCs have, in the past, been used as refrigerants and aerosol propellants. The use of all three of these chemicals has since been restricted or prohibited.[7] Nonetheless, much of the damage that has been done remains.

What Are Direct and Indirect UV Radiation?

Direct UV radiation, or UV radiation that travels from the sun in a straight line, may pose the greatest risk to our health, but we are also at risk from exposure to indirect (scattered and reflected) UV radiation. Scattered UV radiation results from being bounced around by atmospheric dust and water droplets in clouds. Throughout the day, the level of indirect UV radiation varies, as does the level of direct UV radiation. In the early morning and late evening when the sun is low on the horizon, indirect UV radiation may exceed direct. Likewise, on a cloudy day, UV radiation scattered by atmospheric particles may result in greater exposure to indirect than to direct UV radiation.

UV radiation can also be reflected off buildings and the terrain. Smoother surfaces, such as concrete or asphalt, whether they are dark in color or not, typically result in greater reflectance of UV radiation than irregular surfaces. Surface irregularities, such as that found in grass or bark nuggets, reduce the level of reflectance, thereby reducing exposure to reflected UV radiation. One exception, however, is water. Smooth water absorbs almost all UV radiation, whereas the irregular surface of choppy water reflects a considerable amount of UV radiation. The following table lists surfaces and terrains commonly encountered on school grounds and their UV radiation reflectance. Materials with a lower reflectance are more desirable.

How is UV Radiation Measured?

In the past, different countries measured and reported solar UV radiation intensity in different ways. One common way of reporting UV radiation intensity was in the form of estimated "burn time" or "time to burn," expressed as the number of minutes of solar exposure required for the reddening of a fair-skinned person's exposed skin, assuming a clear sky. Although there may be some advantages to this method of reporting UV radiation intensity, there are a number of disadvantages. In 1994, international agreement was reached on standardizing the measure of UV radiation intensity.

Revised by the World Health Organization in 2002 and adopted by the Environmental Protection Agency and the National Oceanic and Atmospheric Administration's National Weather Service in 2004, the UV Index is the internationally accepted system for reporting the intensity of UV radiation. Although the mathematical model developed to determine the UV Index might be complicated, the measurement is easy to understand. The UV Index is a measure of the amount of damaging UV radiation that reaches the earth's surface at noon on a given day and at a given location, expressed as a risk scale. It is predicted daily on a scale of 0 to 11+, where 0 represents a minimal risk of overexposure to UV radiation and any number higher than 11 represents an extreme risk of overexposure to UV radiation.

Ultraviolet Radiation Reflectance for School Grounds Surfaces

Surface	UV Radiation Reflectance[8,9,10]
Grass	1% – 4 %
Still water	3% – 8 %
Soil	4% – 6 %
Asphalt	4% – 9 %
Concrete	7% – 12 %
Choppy water	8% – 13%
Dry sand	15% – 18 %
Fresh snow	85% – 88 %

SHADE PLANNING TOOLBOX

Q: Where do I find the UV Index for tomorrow?

A: In most communities, the UV Index is reported in newspapers and on television with the daily weather forecast.

Every day at approximately 1:30 PM Eastern, the National Oceanic and Atmospheric Administration (NOAA) and the Environmental Protection Agency (EPA) post the UV Index for the next day at the EPA's Website, http://www.epa.gov/sunwise/ uvindex.html.

What Are the Health Effects of Exposure to UV Radiation?

Few people would dispute the beneficial effects of solar radiation. The sun warms the earth, fuels photosynthesis, and ensures the continued existence of life on earth. Many of us enjoy the warmth of the sun on our skin. But at some point in our lives, most of us have experienced the painful effect of too much sun exposure in the form of sunburn. Having experienced sunburn, many would agree that there must be some negative health effect to exposure to the sun. Although many different conditions occur as a normal response to exposure to UV radiation, they all fall into one of two classifications, acute or chronic. Acute effects of UV radiation exposure usually have a rapid onset and are of short duration, such as sunburn, tanning, and synthesis of vitamin D_3. Chronic effects of UV radiation exposure usually have a gradual onset and are of long duration, such as skin cancer and photoaging.

Sunburn

Sunburn is an acute injury resulting from excessive exposure to the sun. The redness associated with sunburn results from the dilation of superficial blood vessels in the skin. Redness usually appears within 4 hours of exposure, reaches a maximum within 12 hours, and fades after a few days. High doses of UV radiation can result in blistering and peeling.

Skin color, hair color, eye color, and freckles all are characteristics that help predict an individual's susceptibility to sunburn. Individuals are typically grouped into one of six sun-reactive types, ranging from those with blue or green eyes and very light skin that never tans to those with very dark hair and eyes and dark skin that almost never burns. Although sunburn is not as common among blacks, compared to whites, blacks are susceptible. Approximately 15% of the African American respondents to a national health survey reported experiencing mild to severe sunburns.[11] Differences also exist in the sun-sensitivity of different parts of the body. The face, neck, and trunk are two to four times more sensitive than the limbs.[12]

Tanning

Tanning, or melanin pigmentation, is a consequence of overexposure to the sun that many people find desirable. UVA exposure results in the skin's production of more melanin, the substance responsible for skin's pigmentation. There are two ways in which our skin can tan, by immediate tanning and by delayed tanning. Immediate tanning occurs as quickly as 5 to 10 minutes after exposure to the sun and will last as long as 2 hours. One's ability to exhibit immediate tanning is directly related to the genetically determined pigmentation of the skin. Delayed tanning, which is the more familiar form of tanning, is noticeable 1 to 2 days after exposure, increases for several days, and lasts for weeks or months. Although having a tan provides some degree of protection from UVB, melanin is not an effective sunscreen for Caucasian skin.[13]

Photosynthesis of Vitamin D_3

The only positive health effect associated with exposure to solar UV radiation is the synthesis of vitamin D_3. Without UVB, the body cannot synthesize vitamin D_3, which is essential for regulating calcium metabolism. Few studies have examined the effect of sun avoidance or the use of sunscreen on the production of vitamin D_3in children or adults. Therefore, the American Academy of Pediatrics has recommended that infants, children, and adolescents who do not consume at least 500 mL (16.9 oz) of vitamin D-fortified milk or formula daily should take one of the many available daily multivitamin supplements that contain 400 IU of vitamin D_3.[14]

Photoaging of the Skin

Exposure to UVA and UVB radiation, and perhaps to radiation in the infrared range as well,[13] causes photoaging, a process in which the skin's elastic fibers break down leading to wrinkled and leathery-looking skin. Dryness, deep wrinkles, sagging, loss of elasticity, and mottled pigmentation are all photoaging symptoms.

Eye Damage

Eye damage from solar radiation is a risk factor for developing a number of eye disorders including cataracts, skin cancer around the eyes and degeneration of the macula. Although the evidence is not conclusive, such damage appears to have a dose-response relationship and to be cumulative; that is, the more unprotected solar radiation exposure to the eyes over an entire lifetime, the greater one's risk for developing cataracts.[13, 15, 16]

Basal Cell Cancer

Typically occurring on the most sun-damaged parts of the body, basal cell carcinoma is a slow-growing cancer that begins as a raised lump on the skin and eventually breaks open to form an exposed sore. Although most of these types of cancers are colorless, some are dark in color. Like other skin cancers, basal cell cancer usually appears in middle age, as a result of UV radiation exposure during childhood or adolescence.

> **SUN PROTECTION IS THE KEY**
>
> The vast bulk of skin cancers in the U.S. are due to excessive skin exposure to UV radiation from the sun, so sun protection is the key to preventing the disease.
>
> Martin Weinstock, MD, PhD Director of Dermatoepidemiology at Brown University and Chair of the American Cancer Society (ACS) Skin Cancer Advisory Board

Squamous Cell Cancer preventing the disease.

Squamous cell cancer is a more aggressive form of skin cancer that ultimately basal cell cancer in appearance. It often follows a pre-cancerous condition called actinic keratosis, which is a dry and crusty area on the skin. Both basal cell and squamous cell carcinoma usually result from chronic exposure to UV radiation over a period of years.

Melanoma

By far, the most serious consequence of exposure to UV radiation is malignant melanoma. Unlike the other two types of skin cancer, basal cell and squamous cell, melanomas involve the dark pigmented cells of the skin, the melanocytes. A growing body of evidence indicates that intermittent sun exposure, as opposed to chronic sun exposure, causes this most deadly of skin cancers. Of particular concern, findings from certain studies point to childhood exposure to sunlight, especially severe childhood sunburn, as an indicator for melanoma as an adult.[17, 18, 19, 20]

Where Can I Find More Information?

Section 5, "The Earth-Sun Relationship," provides more information on seasonal sun angles and their effects on shade design. On the following pages are internet links to more information on skin cancer and its prevention as well as to sun-safety curricula.

Information on Skin Cancer and its Prevention

The Centers for Disease Control and Prevention	
www.cdc.gov/cancer/nscpep/ skin.htm	CDC provides leadership for nationwide efforts to reduce illness and death caused by skin cancer. Although these efforts comprise a variety of approaches and strategies, their common focus is education and prevention. CDC's Web site describes programmatic approaches to skin cancer prevention and education.
The National Cancer Institute	
www.nci.nih.gov/cancertopics/types/ skin	The National Cancer Institute (NCI) is a component of the National Institutes of Health (NIH) and is the federal government's principal agency for cancer research and training. Articles related to the causes of cancer, diagnosis, prevention, treatment, and the most current cancer statistics are available at NCI's Web site.
The United States Environmental Protection Agency	
www.epa.gov/ebtpages/ humasunprotection.html	The Environmental Protection Agency's mission is to protect human health and to safeguard the natural environment. The agency's Web site contains information about the health risks posed by UV radiation and describes the steps people can take to protect themselves from overexposure to the sun.
The National Council on Skin Cancer Prevention	
www.skincancerprevention.org	The mission of the National Council on Skin Cancer Prevention is to facilitate national skin cancer awareness and prevention efforts through education and promotion of sun-safe behaviors. The council, comprising of 30 separate organizations, increases awareness and prevention behaviors among all populations by providing special programs addressing high-risk populations, including infants, children, young adults, parents, educators, outdoor workers, and athletes. Back issues of NEWSLINK, the council's quarterly electronic newsletter, are available at the ogranization's Web site.

The American Cancer Society	
www.cancer.	The American Cancer Society is the nationwide community-based voluntary health organization dedicated to eliminating cancer as a major health problem by preventing cancer through research, education, advocacy, and service. The organization's Web site provides the latest research , information about activities and resources at the local level, and educational and advocacy materials.
The Skin Cancer Foundation	
www.skincancer. org	The Skin Cancer Foundation is the only national and international organization that is concerned exclusively with the world's most common malignancy—cancer of the skin. The foundation's Web site offers information on the three types of skin cancer; information on skin cancer prevention; news of local and national events; and public information posters, pamphlets, and brochures.

Sun Safety Curricula

National Safety Council—Environmental Health Center	
1025 Connecticut Avenue, NW Suite 1200 Washington, DC 20036 www.nsc.org/ehc/sunwise/ activity.htm	The National Safety Council's Enviromental Health Center developed the Sun Safety Activity Guide for elementary school representatives who would like to incorporate sun safety into their school curricula. The guide includes cross-curriculum classroom activities and background information packaged as a 1-hour "core" sun-safety lesson. The core is divided into three 20-minute units, including the effects of UV, risk factors for overexposure to the sun, and sun protection habits. Included in the guide are developmentally appropriate activities for primary (grades K through 2) and intermediate (grades 3 through 6) learning levels.
Project S.A.F.E.T.Y.	
The University of Texas M. D. Anderson Cancer Center with Texas Cancer Council www.mdanderson.org/ departments/ projectsafety/	Project S.A.F.E.T.Y. (Sun Awareness for Educating Today's Youth) is a cross-curricular, multimedia skin cancer prevention program for grades 4 through 9. It is available free of charge to any school in Texas. It is also available to schools outside of Texas for a minimal cost.
The SHADE Foundation	
10510 N. 92nd Street Suite 100 Scottsdale, AZ 85258 www.shadefoundation. org	The mission of The SHADE Foundation, a non-profit organization, is to eradicate melanoma through the education of children and the community in the prevention and detection of skin cancer and the promotion of sun safety. In collaboration with the Environmental Protection Agency (EPA), the Foundation has developed partnerships with schools which implement the EPA SunWise School Program and, in turn, are awarded shade structures to the schools.

Sunny Days, Healthy Ways	
Klein Buendel, Inc. 14023 Denver West Parkway Suite No. 190 Golden, CO 80401 (877) 258-2915 www.info@sdhw.info/	Sunny Days, Healthy Ways is a sun-safety curriculum that uses a comprehensive, cross-curricular approach to teaching skin cancer prevention skills to children in grades K through 5. The curriculum provides an average of 8 hours of sun-safety instruction per grade that can be tailored to the teacher's time frame and needs. The curriculum includes prepared lesson plans, student activity sheets, experiment materials, story books, and assessments.
The SunSafe Project	
Norris Cotton Cancer Center Dartmouth Medical School One Medical Center Drive Lebanon,	The SunSafe intervention aims to enhance and promote sun protection of children ages 2 to 9 years through the delivery of a multicomponent intervention in three settings: elementary schools and day care centers, town beach areas, and primary care practices. The school/day care component consists of an age-specific (2 to 9 years old) and grade-specific curriculum promoting sun protection. Child-care providers and elementary school teachers need 2 theme days or 2 class periods to deliver SunSafe materials. Ongoing reminder activities are suggested as a means for reinforcing the SunSafe message.
The United States Environmental Protection Agency	
SunWise School Program www.epa.gov/sunwise/	The SunWise School Program is an environmental and health education program that aims to teach children and their caregivers how to protect themselves from overexposure to the sun. Using classroom-based, school-based, and community-based components, the SunWise School Program seeks to develop sustained sun-safe behaviors in schoolchildren. The program's learning components build on a solid combination of traditional and innovative education practices already in use in many U.S. elementary and middle schools. Through the program, students and teachers will increase their awareness of simple steps that they can take to protect themselves from overexposure to the sun. Students will demonstrate the ability to practice health-enhancing behaviors and reduce health risks. Children also will acquire scientific knowledge and develop an understanding of environmental concepts related to sun protection. Currently, more than 12,000 schools are registered for the SunWise program, representing all 50 states, the District of Columbia, and Puerto Rico.

Commercial Products Disclaimer

The list of product manufacturers and retailers is provided for general information purposes only and does not represent an inclusive list of vendors. Furthermore, reference to any specific commercial products or services by trade name, trademark, manufacturer, or otherwise, does not constitute or imply its endorsement, recommendation or favoring by the Centers for Disease Control and Prevention (CDC).

The list of product manufacturers and retailers contains URL addresses to Web sites and information created and maintained by private organizations. These links are provided for convenience of reference only. CDC does not control or guarantee the accuracy, relevance, timeliness, or completeness of this outside information. The inclusion of URL addresses to particular Web sites is not intended to reflect their importance, nor is it intended to endorse any views expressed or products or services offered by the author of the site or by the organization operating the server on which the site is maintained.

SECTION 2. STRATEGIES FOR PROVIDING SHADE

A number of strategies for providing shade on school grounds are available; however, no single approach is best for all schools. This section introduces three strategies for providing shade on school grounds: solid roof structures, shade cloth structures, and natural shade. Some of the advantages and disadvantages of each approach are discussed. This information will assist schools in determining how best to provide shade for their students, teachers, staff, and visitors. Regional differences in vegetation, the need for winter warmth, playground usage patterns, and seasonal weather threats to playground structures factor into the decision process of determining the best approach for each school. For many schools, a combination of strategies that capitalizes on the advantages of several approaches will be the most effective.

Solid Roof Structures

Solid roof structures are permanent structures that provide protection from the sun's harmful rays and can be designed to serve a multitude of purposes. Typically, the structures are designed to be open on at least three sides and often include furniture that can be moved around. To maximize flexibility, the design can include lighting and plumbing.

Advantages

- Provides "all-weather" protection.
- Provides additional classroom space.
- Provides exercise space during inclement weather.

- Provides flexibility of design.
- Can be used as a lunch or picnic area.
- Has a long life span.

Disadvantages

- Requires drainage and guttering.
- Can be more expensive than other strategies.

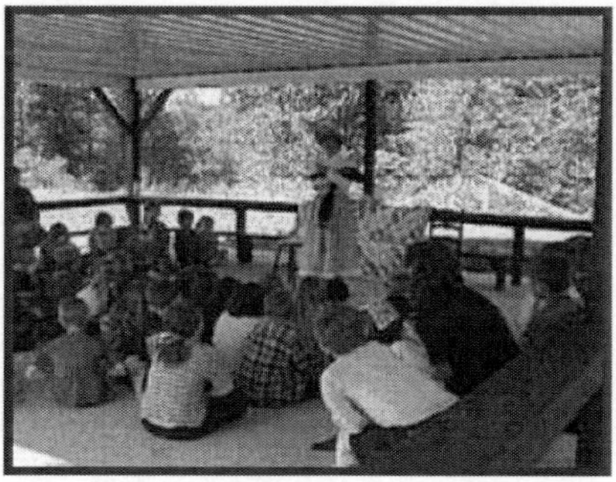

Outdoor classroom at Poplar Creek Elementary School—Siler, Kentucky.

With little more than a few hundred dollars, the support of local businesses, and a State environmental education grant, Principal Tom Shelly and the teachers at Poplar Creek Elementary School, along with the students and their parents, were able to fund the construction of this outdoor classroom and nature trail on their school grounds that otherwise would have cost as much as $30,000.

Considerations

- Schools considering any type of construction project will need to determine which of their local building codes and fire codes are applicable to their project.
- Careful planning will result in the positioning of the structure so that it creates shade at the right place, at the right time of day, throughout the year.
- Schools located in areas that experience heavy snowfall will need to consider the snow load when designing the roof of the structure.
- Likewise, schools located in areas that experience high winds will need to design accordingly.

- Exposed roof supports may be attractive nesting sites for birds. Strategies to deter this should be incorporated into the building's design.
- Lighting will allow for evening use of the building.
- To provide additional light during daytime hours, polycarbonate panels can be incorporated into the roof design and provide a great deal of light while blocking up to 99% of ultraviolet (UV) radiation.

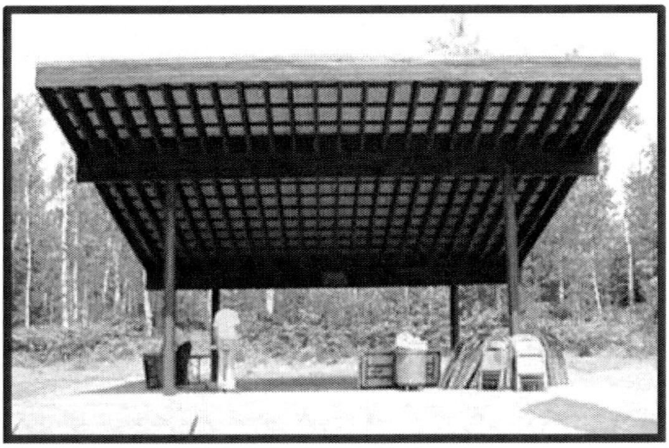

Outdoor classroom at Hermantown School Duluth, Minnesota.

Constructed by the Duluth Skyline Rotary Club as a gift to the Hermantown School District, the outdoor classroom is directly behind the Hermantown Elementary School. Besides serving as an outdoor classroom, the building is accessible to elementary school students during recess periods. According to Fred Majeski, the Superintendent of the Hermantown School District, the building, with its metal framing and roof and concrete floor, would have cost the school well over $25,000 to build, had it not been donated by the Rotary Club.

- No matter what type of design is selected, all buildings require maintenance. A maintenance schedule and estimated costs should factor into the design selection process.
- In the design of the structure, efforts should be made to close off the view of the sky by extending the eaves as far as possible. If the sky can be seen by people under the structure, they are at risk for exposure to indirect UV radiation.

- The design of any structure should ensure access for people with disabilities.
- If the structure is to be used as a classroom or meeting room, the acoustics of the building should also be addressed.

Shade Cloth Structures

Another strategy for providing shade on school grounds is the use of shade cloth or structural fabric supported by a framework or poles. This strategy often is used when the goal is to cover large play areas without employing extensive structural support. Shade cloth is typically a knitted or woven fabric that is rated as to how much sun is blocked. Transmission of the sun's rays through the fabric depends on the tightness of the weave or knit, with more densely woven or knitted fabric blocking out more of the sun's radiation. Fabrics with a looser weave transmit between 50% and 80% of the sun's harmful rays and are typically designed for horticultural applications.

Shade cloth that blocks 80% of solar radiation provides the approximate protective equivalent of sunscreen with a sun protection factor (SPF) of 6.7, whereas shade cloth that blocks 94% of solar radiation provides the approximate protective equivalent of sunscreen with an SPF rating of 15. Shade cloth rated to block 94% of solar radiation is the minimum that schools should consider.

Sun Protection Factor (SPF)

Advantages

- Can be relatively inexpensive to construct.
- Generally requires minimal upkeep.

Disadvantages

- Provides varying UV radiation protection.
- Can be susceptible to weather damage.
- Has a shorter life span than solid roof structures.

Considerations

- Because the UV protection qualities of shade cloth and other structural fabrics vary widely, care should be taken in determining the most appropriate fabric.
- Care must be taken in the positioning of supporting posts so that they do not create a danger to children at play.
- As with any other structure, one of shade cloth should be positioned for maximum sun protection.
- The structural integrity of a fabric structure is related to its curvature and positioning. Structures must be designed to withstand the snow and wind loads that can be expected in their locations.
- The design and installation of these structures should be left to specialists. Names and contact information of organizations that design and install fabric shade structures can be found at the end of this section.

WHAT DOES SPF MEAN?

The common interpretation is how much longer skin covered with sunscreen takes to burn as compared to unprotected skin. Sunscreens can be rated for their protective factor against either UVA or UVB radiation or both. The thickness and thoroughness of application, the type of sunscreen, and the frequency of reapplication factor into whether or not sunscreen delivers the protection for which it is rated.

Natural Shade

Incorporating natural shade into the overall design offers several advantages. The best approach to creating shade is one that provides protection from the sun's harmful radiation during the spring, summer, and fall, yet does not completely block the sun's warmth during winter months. Incorporating deciduous trees, shrubs, and vines into the design provides the seasonal variation in protection that structures alone cannot provide. Likewise, evergreen trees, vines, and shrubs planted alongside structures can serve to block wind in the winter and provide protection from scattered UV radiation during the rest of the year.

Advantages

- Reduces the ambient temperature more so than structures.
- Provides seasonal sun protection.
- Provides low-cost alternatives.
- Improves the aesthetics of the school grounds.
- Provides an opportunity for students to learn about nature.

Disadvantages

- Vegetation takes time to grow.
- Trees can create litter, such as leaves, nuts, and fruits.

Considerations

- There are regional differences in vegetation. Plants native to a particular region have evolved to thrive in the conditions prevalent there. Whenever possible, locally grown native varieties of trees, shrubs, and vines should be used in the design. The United States Department of Agriculture (USDA) Cooperative Extension Service agent in your area can help determine the best species for your design.
- The effectiveness of trees and vines in providing UV radiation protection is directly related to the density of the plant's foliage.
- As a rule of thumb, trees should be planted to the south and west of where you want to shade so they can provide it during the midday and afternoon hours. Section 5, "The Earth-Sun Relationship", gives information on creating shade in the right place at the right time.
- Some plants are poisonous or cause allergic reactions. Other plants can attract bees or have dangerous spikes or thorns. One needs to become familiar with the possible harmful effects of the species that are being considered.
- Trees may interfere with a school's electrical service, plumbing, and drainage systems. Care should be taken that vegetation is not planted where it might later present a threat to the school's utility systems.
- Many trees will not tolerate root compaction, which occurs when foot traffic compacts the soil around the roots of a maturing tree. Several strategies will prevent it, including a temporary fence around the maturing tree or specially designed pavers to absorb the impact of busy feet.
- A short-term or transitional structure can be built to provide shade while the vegetation is maturing.

- The first year after planting vegetation is the most important for ensuring the survival of trees, shrubs, and vines. Plants must be watered at regular intervals if rainfall is inadequate. The USDA Cooperative Extension Service agent in your area can help you determine an appropriate watering schedule.
- Some communities have restrictions on water use that might affect decisions on which plants would be most appropriate.

Where Can I Find More Information?

Section 5, “The Earth-Sun Relationship”, gives more information on providing shade at the right place, at the right time, throughout the year. The following pages contain links to information about selecting trees, vines, and shrubs; sources for plants and products related to natural shade strategies; information on creating natural wildlife habitats; organizations that manufacture and install fabric shade structures; and contact information for the USDA’s Cooperative Extension Service.

WILDLIFE HABITAT CREATION

American Forests: A Tree for Every Child	
www.americanforests.org/resources/	The “A Tree for Every Child” project is a hands-on, flexible environmental education program that allows students to see how practical action can create a better world. The project allows schools to teach students the benefits and rewards of planting trees as part of American Forests’ Global ReLeaf 2000 campaign to plant 20 million trees for the new millennium.
Acorn Naturalists	
P.O. Box 2423 Tustin, CA 92781-2423 Toll Free: (800) 422-8886 http://acornnaturalists.com/store	This organization offers resources for science and environmental educators. Offerings include educator guides, interpretative tools, and books on nature and the environment. An online catalog is available.
Cornell Lab of Ornithology	
159 Sapsucker Woods Road Ithaca, NY 14850-1999 Toll Free: (800) 843-2473 http://birds.	This site describes classroom

Project Wild	
555 Morningside Drive, Suite 212 Houston, TX 77005 Phone: (713) 520-1936 www.projectwild.org	Project Wild provides instructional materials that can be adapted for academic disciplines ranging from science and environmental education to social studies, math, and language arts. Numerous education materials, Web links, and guidebooks are available at this site, including the publication *Wild School Sites: A Guide to Preparing for Habitat Improvement Projects on School Grounds.*
Kidsgardening.com	
National Gardening Association 1100 Dorset Street South Burlington, VT 05403 Toll Free: (800) 538-7476 www.kidsgardening.com	This site is an online source of information and materials for environmental science in the classroom. A keyword-searchable resources directory provides links to regional resources.

RESOURCES FOR NATURAL SHADE SOLUTIONS

United States Department of Agriculture *Cooperative State Research, Education, and Extension Service*	
www.csrees.usda.gov/qlinks/partners/state_partners.html	This site provides links to the county offices of the Cooperative Extension Services system in each state. The Cooperative Extension Services system has field agents assigned to each county. That agent will be able to answer your questions regarding the best species to plant for the application that you are considering; provide you with sources for the trees, shrubs and vines; and offer detailed instructions on the proper way to plant and care for them.
United States Department of Agriculture ***U.S. Forest Service/Urban and Community Forestry***	
www.fs.fed.us/ucf/	The goal of the USDA Forest Service Urban and Community Forestry Program is to provide technical and financial assistance to help improve the livability of cities and communities by managing urban forest resources to promote a healthy ecosystem. This Web site provides links to the regional coordinators.
U.S. Department of Agriculture ***Natural Resources Conservation Service***	
www.plants.	The PLANTS Database provides standardized information about plants of the United States and its territories. The databse includes names, distributional data, species abstracts, characteristics, images, and links to related Web sites with information on the region-specific culture for each species.

(Continued)

Treelink	
www.treelink.org	This Web site provides information, research, and networking for people who work in urban and community forestry. Tips on grant writing and fund-raising are also included.
The National Arbor Day Foundation	
www.arborday.org	The National Arbor Day Foundation helps individuals and groups plant and care for trees and encourages the celebration of Arbor Day to advance global environmental stewardship for the benefit of this and future generations.
The International Society of Arboriculture	
www.treesaregood.com	The International Society of Arboriculture is a worldwide professional organization dedicated to fostering a greater appreciation for trees. The Web site was created to provide the public with quality tree care-related information.
U.S. Environmental Protection Agency ***Landscaping with Native Plants***	
Ariel Rios Building 1200 Pennsylvania Avenue, N.W. Washington,	This Environmental Protection Agency site promotes landscaping with native plants and discusses the environmental benefits of using native plant material. Topics discussed include attracting birds and butterflies and being considerate of local weed laws. *The Wild Ones Handbook* is a compendium of practical information for landscaping with native plants.

SECTION 3. PLANNING FOR SHADE

Planning for shade requires the completion of a series of interrelated tasks. These include convening a planning team, conducting a site audit to determine whether the existing level of shade is adequate, determining the most appropriate strategies if more shade is required; and developing a plan to increase the amount of shade accessible to students, teachers, staff, and visitors. The process can be lengthy, taking as long as 1 year. This section briefly describes each step. In section 6, "How to Conduct a Shade Audit," the reader will find more detailed information on the steps for shade planning.

The Shade Planning Team

It is important for any school undertaking a shade planning project to first identify the stakeholder groups that may have an interest in, or be affected by, the resulting plan. Representatives of these groups should be included on the planning team. For most schools, the stakeholder list would include school administrators, the school nurse, coaches, teachers, students, parents, groups that use the school grounds after hours, and neighbors living adjacent to the school. In addition to stakeholder representatives, the planning team may need to call on professions with expertise in horticulture, landscaping, and architecture. Although it may not be necessary to include such individuals on the planning team, taking the time to identify and recruit them during the earliest stages of the planning process will keep the project moving when their expertise is required. The process will be well served if the goals of the team, the roles and responsibilities of its members, and a method for decision making are determined at the outset. In the course of developing and proposing a shade plan, many decisions will need to be made. One method for decision making that lends itself to a participatory process is decision by consensus.

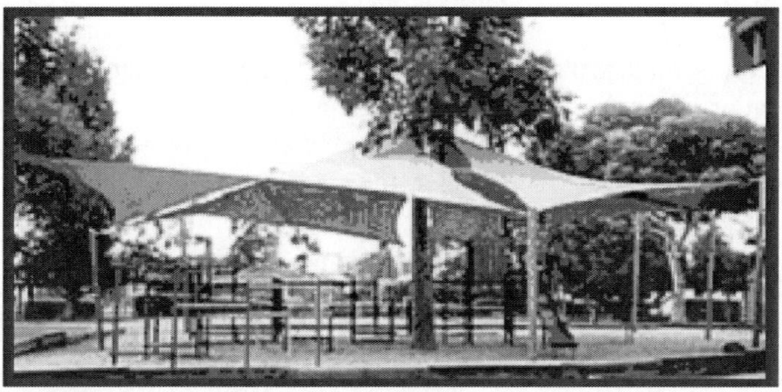

Designed by Shade 'n' Sails of Victoria, Australia.

Transitional shade.

The Shade Audit

Once a planning team has been assembled and its roles, goals, and procedures determined, the group's first major task will be to conduct a shade audit. The audit will help the planning team determine how much shade is currently accessible on the school grounds and if more is needed. The audit consists of a series of user interviews, behavioral observations, and environmental observations. All of the information collected through the audit will be used by the planning group to develop their recommendations.

Interviews

Although members of the planning team may be very familiar with their school, their expertise may not be comprehensive. Any shade planning endeavor should begin by interviewing several members of each of the identified stakeholder groups. In those interviews, the planning team can collect important background information regarding:

- When and where outdoor activities occur.
- Which areas of the school grounds are off-limits.
- Any long-term plans for the school grounds, including new construction.
- Opinions regarding the adequacy of existing shade.
- Expectations regarding the plans for additional shade.

Section 6, "How to Conduct a Shade Audit," contains sample interview questions for school principals, teachers, and students. Planning teams will need to tailor interview questions to issues and concerns specific to their school.

Prior to conducting stakeholder interviews, the planning team should secure a site plan. This is a drawing of the school grounds and buildings that has been drafted to scale. Often site plans are prepared by surveyors or architects, and may be available from the school's principal or the office of the superintendent of the school district. With a site plan, interviewees can refer to activities in relation to the zones and features of the school grounds and interviewers can record the information directly onto the plan.

Behavioral Observations

The next step in the planning process involves collecting data at the school site. Adequate data collection will require several visits to the school. Initial visits will be to observe outdoor activities conducted on the school grounds and document the usage patterns of students, teachers, and staff. Knowing in advance at what times the students can be expected to be outdoors will facilitate the process. Observers will want to document the types of activities taking place, the location in which they are occurring, the number of students participating, and their duration. Once again, it will be helpful for observers to have a site plan on which to make notes regarding outdoor student and teacher activities.

Environmental Observations

Other visits to the site are recommended in order to take measurements on school grounds without interfering with the school's day-to-day activities. On these visits, an accurate site plan will be essential. If none is available, the planning team will need to draw a freehand plan of the site, recording the distances between the various buildings and play equipment. It might be helpful to name different zones if they do not already have names, such as queuing area or passive play area. It is also important to document any significant topographical features, such as low spots, slopes, or ravines, as these will influence decisions about which shade planning strategies will be most appropriate. The site plan should indicate the boundaries of the school's property, which direction is north, and whether it is magnetic north or true north. Often there is an appreciable difference between the two. Determining true north will be important to ensure that shade is cast in the right place, at the right time of day, at the right time of year.

It may also be important to mark the locations of important features outside of the school boundaries, such as the neighboring homes or businesses.

Because ground and building surfaces can reflect ultraviolet (UV) radiation, the planning team should make notes regarding the surfaces and finishes of each building and play area on the school grounds.

It will be important for the planning team to also consider the school's sports areas, such as baseball diamonds, soccer fields, and basketball courts. In thinking about these features of the school grounds, the planning team should take into account the shade needs of the students and coaches who are participating and those of the spectators.

The next task will require some degree of horticultural expertise. The planning team should inventory each tree and planted area on the school grounds. Trees should be numbered on the site plan, and a separate set of notes should record the team's findings for each tree, including the following:

SHADE PLANNING TOOLBOX

When Is North Not Really North?

The short answer is "Almost always!" There is almost always a difference between true north and magnetic north. Fluid motion in the outer core, which is the molten metallic region of Earth, causes the magnetic field to change unpredictably both over time and by location.

Magnetic declination is the measurement of the angle between magnetic north and true north. For example, on July 4, 1955, the magnetic declination for Washington, D.C., was 6 degrees west of true north. On the same day in 2003, the magnetic declination was 10 degrees west of true north.

To find out more about magnetic declination, visit The National Geophysical Data Center at: http://www.ngdc.noaa.gov/seg/ potfld/ declination.shtml

- Species.
- Estimated height.
- Trunk diameter.
- Condition (e.g., broken branches, dead limbs), paying particular attention to any that appear to be unhealthy.
- Estimated diameter of the tree's canopy, that is, the upper part which includes the branches and leaves.
- Density of the tree's canopy.

Notes should also be made on the predominant vegetation for areas of densely planted mixed species.

The final task of the shade audit is to estimate the amount of existing shade on the school grounds. Measurements should be taken of all of the shade, regardless of whether it is in an off-limits area. There are two methods for measuring shade, one of which is highly technical and requires a detailed knowledge of sun projection techniques. The second method requires only that the planning team mark the shade patterns on the ground at the times of day that students are outdoors. The ground can be marked with chalk, rope, or baking flour, then measured and marked to scale on the site plan. Measurements will need to be taken at several times during the day and throughout the school year to ensure that seasonal changes in the shade patterns are recorded.

Assessing the Findings

Having completed interviews with representatives of stakeholder groups, observed usage patterns, and plotted the seasonal shade patterns at the school, the next step in the planning process is to analyze the quantity and quality of shade that is accessible on school grounds, and determine if and where additional shade is needed. The following questions will guide the analysis:

- Will future growth of existing trees result in additional accessible shade?
- Are any areas currently off-limits that could provide additional shade if they were accessible?
- Are any areas protected from direct UV radiation, but not protected from indirect (reflected or diffuse) UV radiation?
- Are there future building plans that might be modified to provide additional shade?

Shade Design

Based on the shade audit, the planning team should present its recommendations in text and graphic format. Recommendations should clearly state the shade goals for each specific zone of the school property, such as bus queuing area, sports venues, active play areas, or informal social gathering places, along with strategies for achieving those goals. The team should consider the range of options at the same time that it is considering the nature of the shade to be provided. Questions that the planning team should take into account when developing a shade plan include:

- Is there a need for protection from rain?
- What are the initial costs for each strategy considered?
- What are the long-term maintenance costs associated with each strategy?
- Is the strategy safe, considering the local weather conditions?
- Is there risk of vandalism, and how can that risk be minimized?

Consulting with knowledgeable architects, landscape architects, or horticulturists is advisable at this point. Not only will they know the species of vegetation that will meet the shade requirements for natural applications and the local building codes for any structural applications, they also can advise the planning team on the potentially complicated tasks of obtaining local building permits and contracting with builders and landscapers.

Funding

At the same time that the planning team is finalizing the shade design, team members can explore potential funding sources and volunteer resources for the project. Several potential sources for funding and hands-on participation are discussed further in section 4, "Case Studies" and in the appendices of this manual. Some possibilities include:

- Contributions from local and national corporations, including in-kind contributions.
- State and federal grants.
- Volunteers and financial contributions from community service organizations.
- Local fund-raisers.
- Support from environmental organizations.
- Advice from local master gardeners associations and programs.
- Volunteer project work for Boy Scout or Girl Scout troops.
- Student class projects.

Where Can I Find More Information?

Section 6, "How to Conduct a Shade Audit," provides more detailed information on the steps of conducting such an audit, including examples of questions that would be appropriate for interviews with stakeholders. On the following pages are resources for facilitating participatory decision-making processes, funding, and working with volunteers.

Resources for Shade Planning Teams

Facilitators Guide to Participatory Decision-Making (1996)	
Sam Kaner, with Lenny Lind, Catherine Toldi, Sarah Fisk, and Duane Berger New Society Publishers Gabriola Island, BC	This guide is designed to help groups increase participation and collaboration; promote mutual understanding; honor diversity; and make effective, inclusive, and participatory decisions.
Evergreen	
355 Adelaide Street West, Fifth Floor Toronto, Ontario M5V 1S2 Phone: (416) 596-1495 www.evergreen.ca	Evergreen is a Canadian non-profit environmental organization with a mandate to bring nature to Canadian cities through naturalization projects. Evergreen motivates people to create and sustain healthy, natural outdoor spaces and gives them the practical tools to be successful. Following are several publications available from Evergreen that should be of interest to shade planning teams. ***Hands for Nature: A Volunteer Management*** *Handbook* This booklet provides practical tips and ideas for working effectively with volunteers to create and sustain greening projects. It includes many insights and helpful statistics from the Community Greening Volunteerism 2002 Survey as well as generous input and discussions with experienced volunteer coordinators and greening participants. ***Design Ideas for the Outdoor Classroom: Dig it, Plant it, Build it, Paint it!*** This booklet is a collection of ideas and techniques for creating native plant and vegetable gardens, and includes a whole range of built and artistic features for your school grounds. ***All Hands in the Dirt: A Guide to Designing and Creating Natural School Grounds*** This manual will guide you through the planning process, providing tips and templates for designing a site that reflects your local natural environment and the ideas of all involved. ***Nature Nurtures: Investigating the Potential of School Grounds*** This report is a comprehensive review of the literature pertaining to school ground naturalization. It examines the work of some of the most advanced thinkers in the fields of child development, education, and environmental psychology, and it explores the web of benefits that results when an entire school community participates in creating more nurturing and diverse environments for learning on the school grounds.

Section 4. Case Studies

Schools and school districts across the United States have already begun the process of shade planning. This section introduces three case studies. The first, Collier County, Florida, demonstrates the power of a single individual to motivate a school board to erect shade canopies over the playgrounds of all of the school district's elementary schools. The second case study, Pinellas County, Florida, demonstrates the fund-raising capacity of schools' parent-teacher organizations (PTOs) and the effect that they can have on decisions of local school boards. Lastly, the story of the collaboration between Shonda Schilling SHADE Foundation and the United States Environmental Protection Agency's SunWise School Program demonstrates the great potential for partnerships that exists for schools and organizations concerned with preventing skin cancer.

Collier County, Florida

Located in Southwest Florida, Collier County encompasses 2,025 square miles and is home to 296,678 residents, according to the U.S. Census Bureau (2004). The January average high temperature is 77.6°, which is also the lowest average high throughout the year. The county's per capita income for the year 1999 was just over $31,000, approximately $3,000 above the U.S. average for that year, and 10.3% of the county's population lived below the U.S. Department of Health and Human Service's poverty guidelines.

One reason for the county's higher-than-average per capita income may be the large number of retirees who have chosen to take up residence in this county. Even with the large percentage of residents older than 65 years of age, almost 20% of Collier County's residents are 18 years old or younger.

The Collier County school district is home to 44 public schools including 2 charter schools. The policy-making body for the school district is a five-member school board.

Getting Started

Teryl Brzeski is a skin cancer survivor. In 1986, at the age of 37, Ms. Brzeski was diagnosed with melanoma, the most deadly form of skin cancer. Her diagnosis motivated her to research the causes of skin cancer and inspired her to do all that she could to help prevent others from developing the disease. "Having a deadly disease and being lucky enough to have a full recovery is a wonderful thing. In my case, it has instilled a passion for being alive and a desire to share cancer prevention information with others."

Ms. Brzeski became especially concerned about her daughter and the other students at Seagate Elementary School. Other Collier County parents were equally concerned about their children's exposure to ultraviolet (UV) radiation. In fact, during the late 1980s, Seagate's PTO raised the $30,000 necessary to erect a pavilion on the school grounds to provide a shaded area for physical education classes. Other than the covered pavilion, however, much of the playground was not protected from excessive solar radiation, and during recess, children played in areas where there was no shade.

Determined to do something about the situation, Ms. Brzeski began her campaign for a shaded playground by researching options for providing shade on school grounds, eventually presenting her ideas to the Collier County School Board. Along with two dermatologists and a representative from the American Cancer Society, she explained to the school board why it was important to provide children, teachers, and staff with adequate protection from solar radiation. Their presentation included an architectural drawing of their vision for a shaded playground at Seagate. Informational packets were distributed to school board members, making a clear and convincing medical case for providing sun protection on a daily basis. The presenters told the school board that they were prepared to raise funds themselves, if necessary, to have the shade structures built.

Approval and Building Costs

The school board not only approved the request for Seagate, but also approved the construction of shade structures on the playgrounds of all Collier County elementary schools at a cost of $2.1 million dollars. In June 2002, Seagate Elementary School became the first county school to be fitted with a shade structure over the playground. By August 2002, before the school year began, 21 more schools in Collier County were fitted with shade structures. Funding for the project was drawn from the school district's capital budget.

Once the school board decided to build the structures, the project was outsourced to a contractor, with specifications that 95% of the playground of each school should be covered by the shade structure. At Seagate Elementary School, the structure covers 8,100 square feet of the playground.

The shade structure comprises multiple canopies. Each canopy is made of a polyethylene mesh fabric that is supported by steel cables and held up by galvanized steel poles, which are secured to concrete pilings. The canopy over Seagate's playground covers a swing set, three slides, and other playground equipment. The polyethylene mesh fabric blocks 90% to 95% of the sun's UV rays. In addition, it allows heat to escape, promoting air circulation. As a result, the temperature beneath the canopies is about 15° lower than that of the ambient air in the middle of the day.

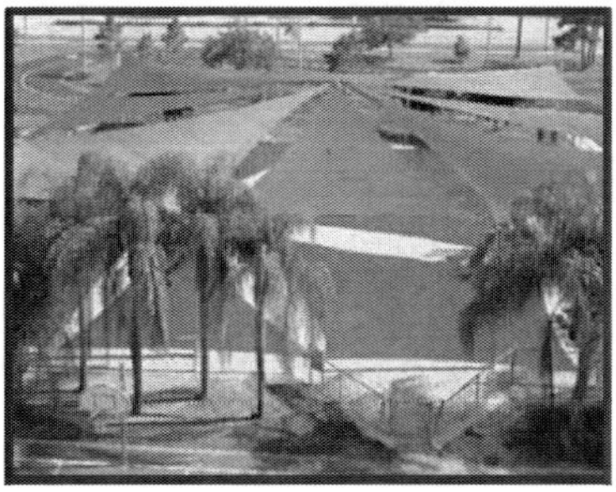

Seagate Elementary School.

Students, teachers, and staff at Seagate Elementary are now protected from ultraviolet radiation during recess.

Maintenance

After the shade structures were built, several potential modifications were identified as necessary to increase the longevity of the structures. For example, additional poles were subsequently added to guard against severe windstorms, and the sails were redesigned and restrung. In 2005 the county incurred additional expenses due to hurricane damage. Consequently, when hurricanes are forecasted, maintenance staff take down the structures. However, contractors must be hired to reassemble them. The county school board will continue their cost benefit analysis and may consider other options in the future.

Continued Efforts

To date, 25 Collier County elementary schools have been outfitted with shade structures over their playgrounds. The scope of the initial project was 22 schools, but since that time, Collier County has built three more schools and has incorporated shade structures into their design and construction.

Since the implementation of shade coverings in the Collier County school district, other neighboring school districts have seen the utility and importance of providing students, teachers, and staff with protection from UV radiation.

For example, in the Lee County school district, Bonita Elementary School has begun fund-raising efforts to build a shade structure for the school. The school's parent-teacher organization has pledged to donate a portion of the funds, and solicitations of businesses and service clubs are expected to raise more. The school expects to pay $64,000 to install shade canopies over its two playgrounds.

Teryl Brzeski has won her battle with skin cancer and now fights every day to ensure that her daughter and the children of Collier County will not have to face the same battle. Her efforts to educate others on skin cancer and its prevention and to promote sun safety through the construction of shade structures at elementary schools have motivated not only her county to take action but have also influenced neighboring counties to take the same steps.

Pinellas County, Florida

Pinellas County, Florida, is located on a peninsula bordered by the Gulf of Mexico and Tampa Bay. The 280-square-mile county is home to about 921,500 year-round residents and welcomes an average of 4.5 million visitors each year. Unemployment in Pinellas County tends to be lower than the Florida state average, which tends to be lower than the national average. According to the U.S. Census Bureau, the per capita income for the year 1999 was just under $24,000, and 12.8% of the county's population lived below the U.S. Department of Health and Human Service's poverty guidelines.

With 114 elementary, middle, and secondary schools, the Pinellas County School District is the 7th largest district in Florida and the 21st largest in the United States.

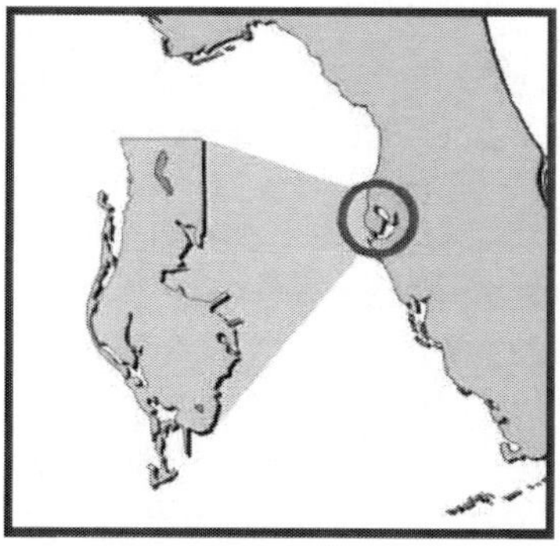

Image source: http://www.pinellascounty.org/.

Getting Started

By 1995, parents and teachers in several of Pinellas County's 82 elementary schools had become concerned about their schools' lack of indoor gymnasium facilities. Physical education classes had to be taught outdoors throughout the year and were canceled when inclement weather required it. The Parent-Teacher Associations (PTA) in those few schools took the initiative to conduct fund-raisers, such as bake sales and jog-a-thons, to collect the $35,000 that each school would need to erect a weather-protected outdoor play area. The schools tapped local expertise in determining the best design for the structures and for executing the construction.

In 2002, the local PTA efforts in Pinellas County paid off for all elementary school children in the county, prompting the Pinellas County school board to determine that all 82 elementary schools in the county should have similar structures to protect students, teachers, and staff. Walter Miller, associate superintendent of institutional services, cites health and medical concerns as the rationale for the school board's decision, "We ensure that the students, faculty, and staff have a clean and safe environment inside of the school, so it's only right that we are concerned about the environment outside of the school as well. Children and physical education teachers were exposed to extreme heat and put at risk for skin cancer, which in Florida is a major concern, so the shade structures buy students and teachers the opportunity to escape the heat and exposure to ultraviolet radiation."

Building Costs

Funding for the construction has been supported through the school district's capital budget. The school district's facilities department identified a general contractor to oversee construction of the buildings, and the contractor received bids from a number of manufacturers. A local firm was ultimately selected, because using a local builder would reduce shipping and travel costs.

To reduce costs, a single design was used for all schools, although each school determined the placement of its shade structure. The structures are 40-by-80 feet, roughly the size of a tennis court, and are constructed of metal with concrete floors. The designers had to consider the threat of strong winds associated with hurricanes or tornados, very real threats in Florida. As a result, a larger foundation was incorporated into the design to create uplift resistance in the event of a windstorm. Each structure approximately cost $60,000, which according to the director of facilities was considerably lower than it would have been if each building had been individually bid. Those schools that had begun fund-raising efforts for a shade structure were allowed to add that money to the school board's budget, and make improvements to the original design, including a larger structure, if that was what the school wanted.

Maintenance

As the oldest of the buildings begin to age, some of the maintenance requirements are becoming more obvious. Most apparent is the need to paint the steel structures regularly to prevent premature rusting. Structures that need repainting must first be sandblasted to remove old paint and rust. In some cases, as more time passes, other maintenance issues will be identified. Recently, some of the schools have experienced problems with birds nesting in the metal framing that supports the roof. Modifications to the design of future buildings and to those already constructed may solve that problem.

Continued Efforts

Currently, 66 of the 82 elementary schools in Pinellas County have shade structures. The school district expects that all schools in the county will have these structures by 2007. This tremendous accomplishment is the result of the efforts of just a few concerned parents, teachers, and principals who recognized the importance of providing sun protection to their students, teachers, and staff.

If you would like to find out more about the efforts to prevent skin cancer at Pinellas County Schools, feel free to contact:

Walter Miller, Associate Superintendent, Institutional Services in Pinellas County Phone: (727) 547-7167

Jim Ewbank, Supervisor of Pre-K Physical Education Phone: (727) 588-6078

SHADE Foundation of America and the U.S. Environmental Protection Agency's SunWise School Program

SHADE Foundation of America

In February 2001, Shonda Schilling, a 33-year old mother of four young children and wife of Boston Red Sox pitcher Curt Schilling, was diagnosed with melanoma. Having been a lifelong sunbather, Ms. Shilling felt a need to inform the public about the dangers of exposure to the sun's UV rays. She learned that although Arizona has the highest melanoma rate in the United States, the state had no organizations devoted to preventing the cancer. As a way to fill that gap, Shonda founded the SHADE Foundation.

SHADE Foundation of America is a non-profit organization dedicated to the education, prevention, and detection of skin cancer. Created in September 2002, the foundation's goal is to prevent the development of skin cancer through educational programs and free skin cancer screenings.

The U.S. Environmental Protection Agency's SunWise School Program

First piloted in May 1999, the SunWise School Program, developed by the United States Environmental Protection Agency (EPA), is an environmental and health education program designed to teach children and their caregivers how to protect themselves from overexposure to the sun. The standards-based, cross-curricular lessons in the SunWise Tool Kit were designed to foster sun-safe behaviors in children and to increase their knowledge and appreciation of the environment. In addition, the program encourages schools to create shade structures, adopt sun-safe policies, and develop additional community partnerships.

Since the year 2000, the K–8 curriculum has been available on a national basis, free of charge, to any school To participate in the SunWise program, schools must adopt a SunWise activity, which may include implementing classroom lessons, collecting and reporting UV radiation data, adopting school-wide sun-safe policies, or engaging in skin cancer prevention community outreach. Schools must also participate in a program evaluation.

Creating a Collaboration

The development of the collaboration between the SHADE Foundation and the EPA began in October 2002. Linda Rutsch, Director of the SunWise School Program at the EPA, was visiting the Web site of a melanoma foundation in Nevada when she noticed a link to the SHADE Foundation. "Usually I will check out various links in order to keep up with what's out there," Ms. Rutsch recalls. She clicked on the SHADE Foundation's link, learned about the Foundation's skin cancer prevention efforts in Arizona, and found a contact name. Ms. Rutsch called Sue Gorham, executive director of the SHADE Foundation, and told her, "I would like to send you a SunWise Kit and tell you a little about our program."

As luck would have it, the SHADE Foundation was in the process of searching for a school curriculum on sun safety. Ms. Schilling and Ms. Gorham decided to develop a program for schools that would allow them to acquire shade structures for their campuses through the SHADE Foundation. The idea was to encourage schools to implement a sun-safe curriculum and to develop sun-safe policies within the school.

The EPA's SunWise curriculum was exactly what the SHADE Foundation was seeking, and the partnership began there. As Ms. Rutsch remembers, "That was in October of 2002 when we first started corresponding. In January of 2003, we had our first face-toface meeting where we talked about working together."

How the Program Works

The **SHADE SunWise School Program** requires schools to qualify in two steps. The first step is to request the EPA SunWise curriculum, usually via the EPA SunWise Web site. Once a school has reviewed the curriculum and made the decision to implement it, the next step is to apply to the SHADE Foundation to participate in the SHADE SunWise School Program. The written grant statement must include a description of the policy and activities the school proposes to adopt for skin cancer prevention. Upon demonstration of sustained teaching activities and the implementation of sun protection policies, the Foundation gives grants for the consideration of a shade structure.

The shade structures are an appropriate reward for the school's achievements. Besides protecting students, teachers, staff, and visitors from overexposure to UV radiation, the structures contribute to a more comfortable environment for students to enjoy outdoor physical activities. As Sue Gorham points out, "Here in Arizona, when children slide down the sliding board, it is so hot that it could take the skin off their backs. Under these shade structures, the temperatures will drop as much as 20 degrees."

Building Costs

The cost for providing a school with the 24' x 35' shade structure is between $6,000 and $10,000. The shade structures are of shade cloth, approximately 24' x 35' and hoisted on metal poles. The shade cloth provides 98% protection from UV radiation. Schools have flexibility in determining where on their grounds would be the most appropriate location for their shade structure.

The SHADE Foundation assumes all costs of the shade structures, with money raised through a number of fund-raising events, ranging from auctions to golf tournaments. The first year of implementation was used to demonstrate both the program's needs and SHADE's fiscal responsibility and ability to execute the managerial and administrative duties of the project. Hoping to supplement its fund-raising efforts with grant money, the program began applying for grants in 2004. In 2005, SHADE received its first grant of $25,000 from Teammates for Kids. SHADE, now in its 4th year of giving grants, has funded approximately 50 structures across the nation at a cost of $267,000.

Though some schools have expressed concern over the required maintenance on the structures, to date this has not been a great problem, because the structures have not required much maintenance.

Continued Efforts

To date, the SHADE Foundation has constructed 50 shade structures in U.S. schools and community areas which benefit children. In the coming year, the Foundation plans to raise funds to support 95% of grant applications.

The SHADE Foundation and EPA were recognized for their work by being awarded the "2003 Excellence in Cancer Awareness Award," presented by Congressional Families Action for Cancer Awareness. This award is presented annually to the organization that best exemplifies a total commitment and dedication to assisting others in preventing cancer. This award honors the partnership between the SHADE Foundation and the EPA SunWise program in addressing the issue of skin cancer prevention. "We are so proud of our partnership receiving the award," says Ms. Gorham. "We hope that through qualifying for grants in the future, we will be able to carry on this work in all states."

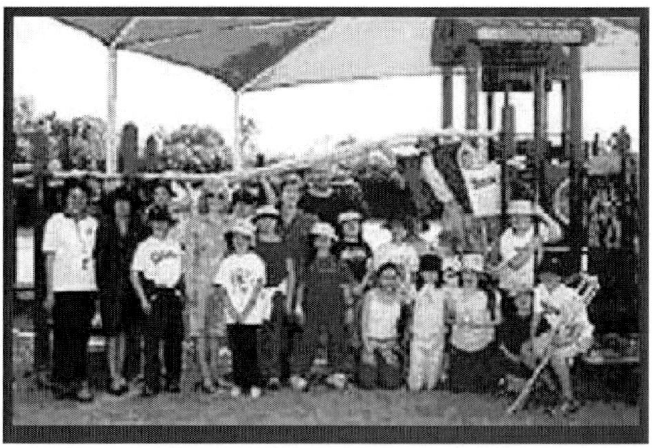

Cherokee Elementary school: the first school to graduate with the SHADE Foundation and SunWise curriculum.

If you would like to find out more about the SHADE Foundation's efforts to prevent skin cancer, feel free to contact:

Sue Gorham Executive
Director of the SHADE Foundation
www.shadefoundation.org
Phone: (480) 614-2278
Fax: (480) 614-2279
E-mail: sue@shadefoundation.org
To find out more about the EPA's SunWise School Program, contact:
Linda Rutsch
Director of the SunWise Program
www.epa.gov/sunwise
Phone: (202) 343-9924
Fax: (202) 343-2362
E-mail: rutsch. linda@epa.gov

Key Terms and Concepts

Latitude is a north-south measurement of any position on the Earth. Measured in degrees, latitude is 0° at the equator and 90° at the North and South Poles. The line that connects all locations of the same latitude is called a parallel. Shade planning teams will need to know the latitude to determine where a tree or structure will cast its shadow throughout the day.

Longitude is a west-east measurement of any position on the Earth. The line that connects all locations of the same longitude is called a meridian. Longitude, like latitude, is measured in degrees, with 0° occurring at the Greenwich Meridian or Prime Meridian. Measurements of longitude range from Prime Meridian at 0° to 180° going either west or east. The 180th meridian east is the International Date Line. Shade planning teams will need to know their longitude to determine solar noon.

Solar Noon is the time of day when the sun is aligned with true north and true south and is specific to each longitude. In the northern hemisphere, a shadow cast by a vertical pole at solar noon will point toward true north. Solar noon is also the midpoint between sunrise and sunset.

Section 5. The Earth-Sun Relationship

For any shade planning team, the primary objective is to ensure that shade falls in the right place, at the right time of day, throughout the year. A shade planning team should include members with at least a working knowledge of the Earth's relation to the sun. This section is designed to:

- Graphically illustrate the effects of daily and seasonal changes in solar angles on the length and direction of shadows.
- Provide a basic introduction, or reintroduction, to the Earth's relationship to the sun and solar geometry.
- Provide a list of resources that can assist the planning team in ensuring that shade falls in the right place, at the right time of day, throughout the year.

The Sun's Annual Path and the Creation of Shade

Shadows cast by the sun grow longer from June 21st until December 21st, and then grow shorter from December 21st until June 21st. This is a result of annual changes in the solar altitude angle. The change in shadow length is depicted graphically in the following illustration. A 36-foot tall tree with a canopy spread of 48 feet planted at the geographic center of the contiguous United States (Longitude=98°3'West; Latitude=39°0'North) tree would cast shadows at **solar noon** throughout the year as follows:

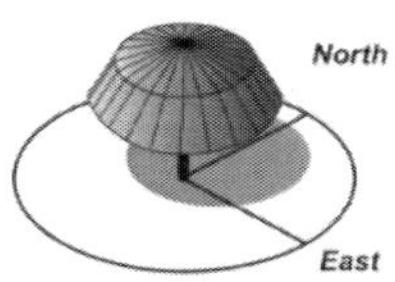

August 21

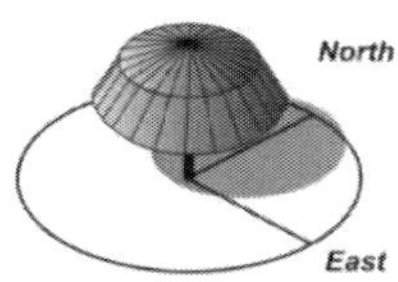

September 21

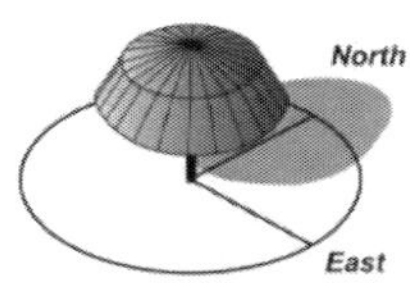

October 21

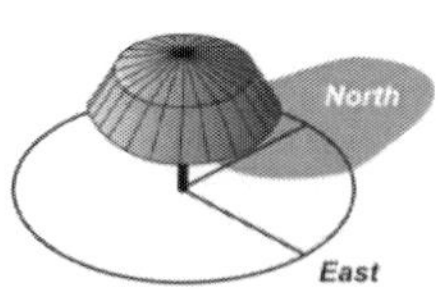

November 21

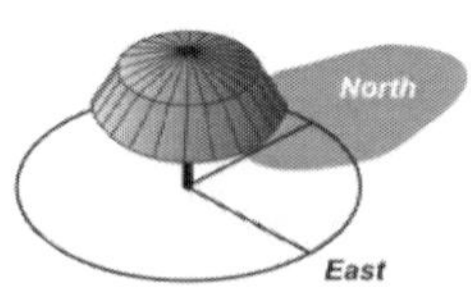

December 21

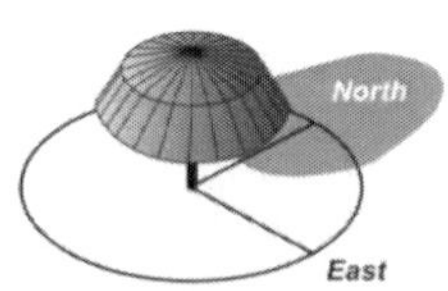

January 21

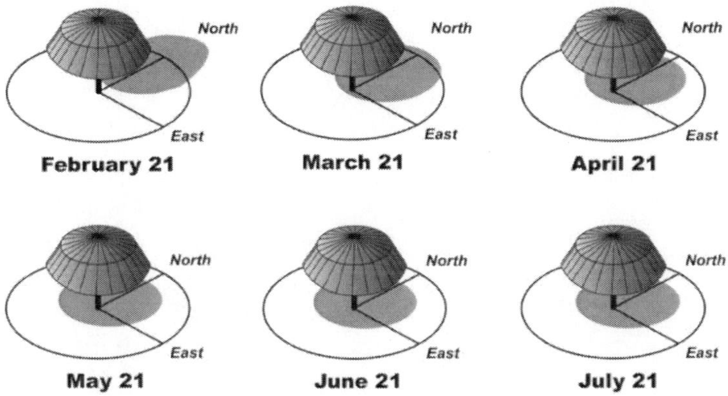

The Sun's Daily Path and the Creation of Shade

Observing that same 36-foot tall tree, the shadows that are cast move from west to east throughout the day in response to the sun's east-to-west movement. On March 21st, the shadows that would be cast throughout the school day would appear as follows:

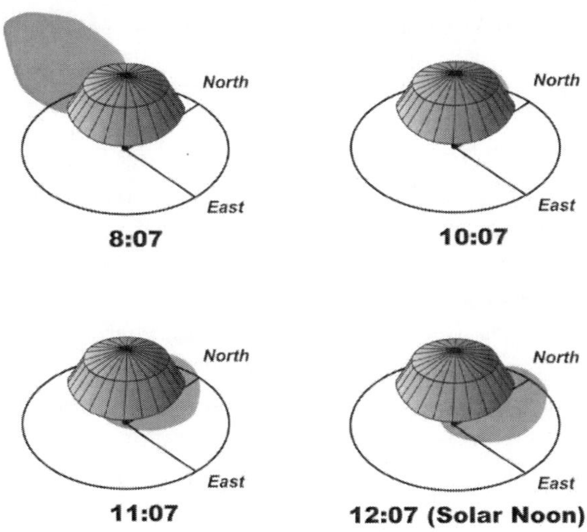

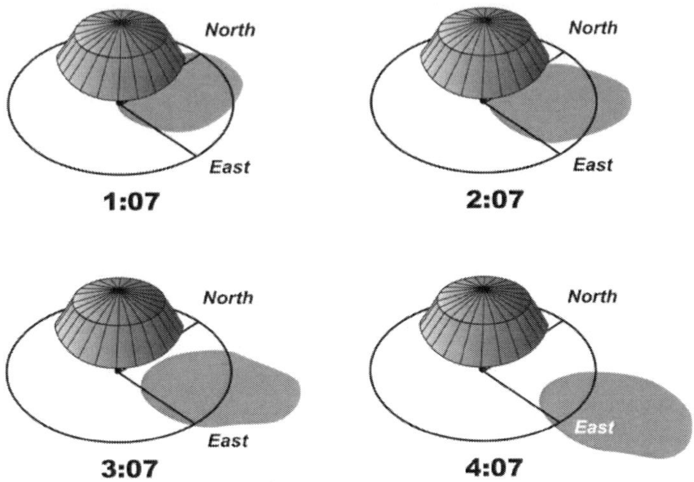

The Earth's Rotation and Revolution

Every 24 hours, the Earth makes one rotation on its axis; every 365.24 days, the Earth makes one revolution around the sun. If one were to view the Earth spinning on its axis, one would note that the axis is not perpendicular to the Earth's orbit around the sun, but is tilted at an angle of 23.5°, with the North Pole always pointing directly at the North Star. Furthermore, the Earth's orbit around the sun is not circular, but elliptical, causing the Earth's distance from the sun to vary by as much as 3 million miles throughout the year. The annual variation in the Earth's distance from the sun affects the amount of solar radiation intercepted by the Earth by as much as 7%. The changing distance from the sun, however, is not responsible for the changes in seasons. The changes in season are caused instead by the constant 23.5° tilt of the Earth and the Earth's rotation around the sun.

Summer solstice, which is on or about June 21st, marks the beginning of summer in the northern hemisphere. The Earth is positioned so that the North Pole is leaning toward the sun at 23.5°. On summer solstice, the length of the day, from sunrise until sunset is greater than 12 hours for all latitudes north of the equator, and less than 12 hours for all latitudes south of the equator. On summer solstice, the center of the sun lines up with the latitude known as the Tropic of Cancer, which is at 23.5° north.

KEY TERMS AND CONCEPTS

The Earth's axis of rotation is not perpendicular to its orbit around the sun, but is tilted at an angle of approximately 23.5°. **Solar Declination** is the angle that a given hemisphere is tilted toward the sun on any given day. It is marked by the latitude on the Earth where the location of the sun is directly overhead at solar noon. Because of the 23.5° tilt, this location is always somewhere between 23.5° north and 23.5° south, depending on the time of the year. Solar declination is 0° when the sun lines up with the equator on the equinoxes.

Equinox is one of the two periods when the declination of the sun is 0°, or the sun is lined up exactly with the equator. The autumnal equinox occurs on or about September 21st, and the vernal equinox occurs on or about March 22nd. Only on these 2 days are the hours of the day and night equal, and only on these 2 days does the sun rise due east and set due west.

Solstice is either the longest or the shortest day of the year. In the northern hemisphere, summer solstice is the longest day of the year and occurs on or about June 21st. Winter solstice occurs on or about December 22nd.

True north, also known as geographic north, is the northernmost point on the Earth as determined by the Earth's rotation. This usually differs from what a compass indicates as north. When a compass points to north, it is pointing toward magnetic north, which in some locations in the United States, may be as far as 20° from true north.

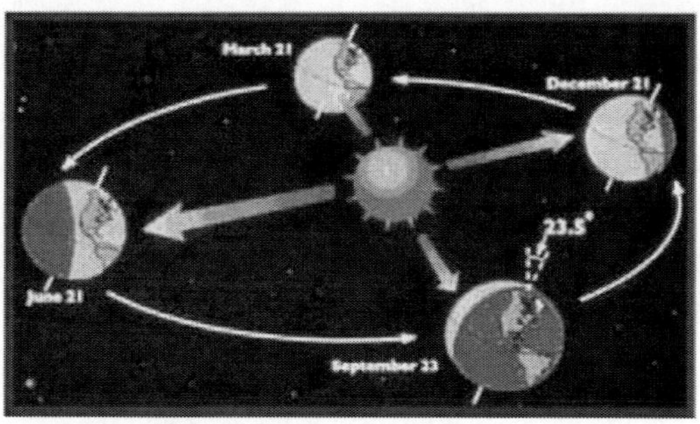

Image Source: National Geophysical Data Center.

At the winter solstice, on or about December 22nd, the Earth is positioned so that the North Pole is leaning away from the sun, and all latitudes south of the equator experience days longer than 12 hours and all latitudes north of the equator experience days shorter than 12 hours. This marks the beginning of summer in the southern hemisphere and the beginning of winter in the northern hemisphere. On winter solstice, the center of the sun lines up with the latitude known as the Tropic of Capricorn, which is at 23.5° south.

On the equinoxes, those being around September 21st and March 21st, the Earth is positioned so that the North Pole points neither toward nor away from the sun. On those 2 days, the Earth's equator lines up with the center of the sun, resulting in days that are exactly 12 hours long, regardless of latitude.

KEY TERMS AND CONCEPTS

Solar azimuth angle is the angle on the horizontal plane between the point on the horizon that is directly beneath the sun and true south. The azimuth angle determines the direction of shadows.

Solar elevation angle or solar altitude angle is the angle that describes the height of the sun in relation to the nearest point on the horizon. It varies according to the time of day and the season and determines the length of shadows.

Axis Tilt and Solar Radiation

That the Earth's axis is tilted affects the amount of solar radiation reaching the Earth in three ways. First, the length of the day changes throughout the year. In the northern hemisphere, beginning on the summer solstice, the sun's daily path is increasingly lower in the sky (making shadows longer) until the winter solstice, after which the days become increasingly longer. As days grow longer, the risk of exposure to excessive ultraviolet (UV) radiation is greater.

Second, when the sun is at a lower altitude, its rays are spread over a larger area, reducing the intensity of the sun's radiation, including UV radiation.

Third, levels of solar radiation are also affected by how much of the atmosphere the sun's rays must pass through. Solar radiation levels, including UV radiation, are greatest when the sun is higher in the sky and solar radiation has a shorter path to travel through the atmosphere. When the sun is lower in the sky, solar radiation has a longer path to travel through the atmosphere, resulting in more of the sun's radiation, including UV radiation, being absorbed or scattered by the atmosphere.

Putting It All Together

In order to create shade that falls in the right place, at the right time of day, throughout the year, it is essential that the planning team model the shade that their proposed buildings and plantings will cast. To do that, the team will need to know:

- Longitude and latitude of the school's location.
- Location of true north and true south.
- Size, shape, and orientation of proposed buildings.
- Growth patterns and locations of proposed plantings.
- Time of day that solar noon occurs throughout the year at that longitude.

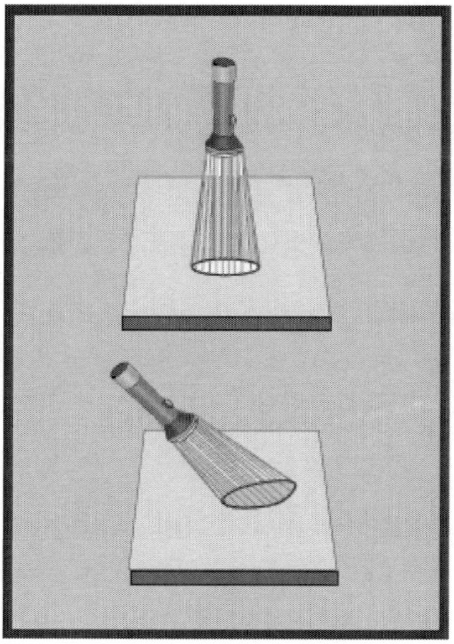

The more perpendicular a beam is to a surface, the brighter the beam will be on the surface.

Armed with that information and a working knowledge of solar geometry, it is possible to use mathematical and geometrical procedures to model the shade that will be cast by proposed structures and plantings. A number of computer software programs are available to do that work for you. Following are descriptions of two such programs, one of which has been developed for modeling sun and shade patterns for solar collectors, though it may well fit into the budgets and serve the purposes of some schools. The other is a program that has been designed specifically for shade planning.

Visual Sun Chart

www.visualsunchart.com/

Visual Sun Chart is a graphics program that was developed for visualizing solar shading to maximize the efficiency of solar collectors. It allows the user to model trees and buildings and, along with a free download, visualize the shade patterns that are cast. With Visual Sun Chart, a user can:

- Model buildings and trees.
- Export scenes to POV Ray 3.5, a free download that models shade produced by buildings and trees.
- Create reports which give information about positions of the sun, times of sunrise and sunset, horizontal and vertical shadow angles, and angles of incidence.
- View and print 3D models of sun movements.

webShade

www.shadeaudit.com.au
www.webshade.com.au

webShade is an interactive software package that allows users to prepare shade audits without the need for technical skills or expertise. Users can either scan their site plan into the computer or use a simple drawing program to create a 3D model of their site. On completion of the shade audit with webShade, the program produces a printed site plan, complete with shade solutions and simulated outcomes. Available as an internet download, a webShade user can:

- Project existing summer and winter shade patterns.
- Model alternative shade strategies.

- Project the summer and winter shade patterns for those alternatives.
- Prepare presentation-ready materials, including site-specific UV radiation information and design strategies.

Where Can I Find More Information?

To determine a location's latitude and longitude:

- www.pbs.org/wgbh/nova/longitude/find.html
- http://zipinfo.com/search/zipcode.htm
- http://geonames.usgs.gov/pls/gnis/web_query.gnis_web_query_form
- http://tiger.census.gov/cgi-bin/mapbrowse-tbl

To determine the time of day that solar noon occurs:

- http://www.srrb.noaa.gov/highlights/sunrise/sunrise.html
- http://users.vei.net/pelican/sunrise.html
- http://www.spot-on-sundials.co.uk/calculator.html

For more information on solar geometry:

- http://www.geog.ouc.bc.ca/physgeog
- http://education.gsfc.nasa.gov/experimental/July61999siteupdate/inv99Project.Site/ Pages/solar.insolation.html

SECTION 6. HOW TO CONDUCT A SHADE AUDIT

The purpose of the shade audit is to document the usage patterns of the school grounds and determine the amount and quality of existing shade. All of the information collected through the shade audit will be used by the planning group to develop recommendations for making the best use of existing shade and, if required, for creating additional shade. The final product of a shade audit is a written report or presentation of the shade team's findings and recommendations to the school community.

The process includes a series of interviews, behavioral observations, and environmental observations followed by an assessment of the findings and the generation of prioritized recommendations for achieving the goals. The entire process may take as long as 1 year. The first step in the process is to conduct stakeholder interviews.

Stakeholder Interviews

Before the first interview is conducted, the shade planning team should produce a comprehensive list of stakeholder groups that may have an interest in, or be affected by, the resulting plan. The team should identify and invite representatives from each stakeholder group to be interviewed. Ideally, each of the stakeholder groups will be represented on the planning team; nonetheless, it will be necessary to interview members of all stakeholder groups even if they are also represented on the team. For many schools the list would include:

- School administrators.
- Teachers, particularly the physical education teacher.
- Coaches.
- School nurse.
- Students.
- Building maintenance staff.
- Organizers of little league programs or others who may use the school grounds on weekends.
- Residents of the neighborhood adjacent to the school.

Interview Guides

For each stakeholder group, the shade planning team should generate a list of appropriate questions to explore in the interview process. Questions should cover topics with which the interviewee is very familiar. Some may ask the interviewee to discuss outdoor activities that they observe or in which they participate. In order to get the most out of the interviews, interviewers should ask interviewees to reference the school's site plan while describing those activities. This is a scaled drawing of the school grounds and buildings. Often such plans are prepared by surveyors or architects, and may be available from the school's principal or the office of the superintendent of the school district. Referring to a site plan during the interview process allows interviewees to reference activities in relation to the zones and features of the school grounds and allows interviewers to record the information directly onto the site plan. Through the interview process, interviewees may identify school grounds users of whom the shade planning team was not previously aware. Such newly identified stakeholders should be added to the list of interviewees.

Following are examples of questions that would be appropriate for school principals, teachers, students, and other stakeholders. This is not meant to be a comprehensive list, but instead gives samples of questions that might be most appropriate for each stakeholder group. The planning team will need to tailor their questions to the issues and concerns specific to their schools.

Sample Questions for School Principals

- How many students attend the school?
- What is the age range and distribution of the students?
- Does the school have sun-safe policies in effect?
    - Hats?
    - Sunglasses?
    - Long-sleeved shirts?
    - Sunscreen?
- What are the outdoor activities in which students participate?
    - Recess?
    - Lunch?
    - Assemblies?
    - Physical education?
    - Educational activities?
    - Informal social gatherings?
    - Extended day activities?

  Intermural and intramural athletic events?
- For each: Where do they occur? (Have interviewee refer to site plan.)
    - At what time of day do they occur?
    - What is the duration of the activity?
- Do you believe there is adequate accessible shade on the school grounds? If not, where is additional shade most needed? (The interviewee should be asked to refer to the site plan.)
- Is there inaccessible shade on the school grounds that could be made accessible?
- Is there a need for an area on the school grounds that is protected from precipitation?

- Are there plans for making improvements to the school, such as remodeling, adding classroom space, or landscaping projects?
- Does the school currently have problems with, or has it recently experienced problems with vandalism?
- Are there groups that have permission to use the school grounds after school hours and on weekends?
- Are there groups that, without formal permission, use the school grounds after school hours and on weekends?
- Can you think of any barriers to providing additional shade at this school?
- What type of shade do you think would work best at this school (solid-roof structure, shade cloth structure, or natural shade)?

Sample Questions for School Teachers

- What age group do you teach and how many students are in your class?
- What are the outdoor activities in which your class participates?
  - Recess?
  - Lunch?
  - Assemblies?
  - Physical education?
  - Educational activities?
  - Informal social gatherings?
  - Extended day activities?
  - Intermural and intramural athletic events?
- For each: Where do they occur? (Have interviewee refer to site plan.)
  - At what time of day do they occur?
  - What is the duration of the activity?
- Does the school have sun-safe policies in effect?
  - Hats?
  - Sunglasses?
  - Long-sleeved shirts?
  - Sunscreen?
- Do you believe there is adequate accessible shade on the school grounds? If not, where is additional shade most needed? (The interviewee should be asked to refer to the site plan.)

- Is there inaccessible shade on the school grounds that could be made accessible?
- Is there a need for an area on the school grounds that is protected from precipitation?
- Are there times that teachers are required to be outdoors, such as to monitor the activities on the school grounds? If so, how often does this happen and for how long?
- If there were outdoor classroom space, would you use it? Do you think that other teachers would?
- Can you think of any barriers to providing additional shade at this school?
- What type of shade do you think would work best at this school (solid-roof structure, shade cloth structure, or natural shade)?

Sample Questions for Students

- How old are you?
- When you are outside, do you usually play/socailize in the sun or in the shade?
    - During recess?
    - During and after lunch?
    - During physical education class?
    - During extended day activities (if applicable)?
    - Intermural and intramural athletic events (if applicable)?
- For each, where do you play? (Have student refer to site plan.)
- Does the school have sun-safe policies in effect?
    - Hats?
    - Sunglasses?
    - Long-sleeved shirts?
    - Sunscreen?
- Do you believe there is adequate accessible shade on the school grounds? If not, where is additional shade most needed? (The interviewee should be asked to refer to the site plan.)
- Are there shaded areas on the playground that you would prefer not to use? Why?
- Are there areas on the school grounds where you are not allowed to play?

Sample Questions for Building Maintenance Engineers

- Do you believe there is adequate accessible shade on the school grounds? If not, where is additional shade most needed? (The interviewee should be asked to refer to the site plan.)
- Is there inaccessible shade on the school grounds that could be made accessible?
- Is there a need for an area on the school grounds that is protected from precipitation?
- Are there plans for making improvements to the school, such as remodeling, adding classroom space, or landscaping projects?
- How would a plan to plant trees or build a shade structure be affected by the school's utility services? (On the site plan, have the interviewee mark the service lines for the school's utility services.)
- Does the school currently have problems with, or has it recently experienced problems with vandalism?
- Are there groups that have permission to use the school grounds after hours and on weekends?
- Are there groups that, without formal permission, use the school grounds after school hours and on weekends?
- Can you think of any barriers to providing additional shade at this school? For example, would watering trees or removing tree litter be a problem?
- What type of shade do you think would work best at this school (solid-roof structure, shade cloth structure, or natural shade)?

Sample Questions for Neighbors

- Do you believe there is adequate accessible shade on the school grounds? If not, where do you believe that additional shade is most needed? (The interviewee should be asked to refer to the site plan.)
- Do residents of the neighborhood utilize the school grounds for activities on weekends or after school hours?
- In what types of activities have you seen neighbors participate on the school grounds?
- For each: Where do they occur? (Have interviewee refer to site plan.)

On what days of the week and at what time of day do they occur? What is the duration of the activity?

- Is there a need for a rain-protected area on the playground?
- Do you think that the school currently has problems with, or has recently experienced problems with vandalism?
- Can you think of any barriers to providing additional shade at this school?
- If the school were to plant additional shade trees, are there areas on the school grounds where planting them might create a problem for neighbors?
- If the school were to build a shade structure, would it create a problem for neighbors?
- Are there areas of the school grounds where a shade structure might create a problem for neighbors?
- What type of shade do you think would work best at this school (solid-roof structure, shade cloth structure, or natural shade)?

Once all interviews have been conducted, the planning group should meet to discuss their findings. Information collected from different stakeholder sources should be synthesized and clarifications on, or answers to, any resulting questions should be sought by the group.

Behavioral Observations

The next step in conducting a shade audit involves observation of students, teachers, staff, and visitors on school grounds. Visits to school grounds after hours and on weekends will be necessary to confirm non-school–related activities that might be affected by the shade plan. Information collected in the interview process should guide the behavioral observations. Observers will want to document the types of activities, their locations, the number of individuals who participate in each activity, and the duration of the activity. Once again, it will be helpful for observers to make notes regarding all activities on a site plan. Participants in this process should model good sun-protective behaviors by wearing sunglasses, hats, and long-sleeved shirts.

Observations should be made on several occasions to capture the many activities that occur on school grounds and, as much as possible, observations should be made unobtrusively. Observers should note whether activities are occurring in a particular location because no other area will accommodate that activity, or if there are other locations where the activity could take place, particularly a shaded area.

Once again, upon completion of this step, the planning team should meet to discuss findings. If there are discrepancies between the information collected in the interview process and the behavioral observations, the team should note the discrepancies and seek clarification.

Environmental Observations

Other visits to the site will need to be planned to take measurements on school grounds without interfering with the day-to-day activities of the school. On these visits, having an accurate site plan will be essential. If none is available, the planning team will need to draw a freehand plan of the site, taking careful measurements of the buildings and recording the location and size of each. The site plan should indicate the boundaries of the school's property, which direction is north, and indicate if it is magnetic or true north, since there is an appreciable difference between the two. Determining true north will be important to ensure that shade is cast in the right place, at the right time of day, throughout the year. (See text box on page 22 of this manual.)

It may also be important to mark the locations of important features outside of the school boundaries, such as the location of neighboring homes or businesses and any buildings not on school property that cast shadows or reflect solar radiation onto the school grounds.

Once at the site, the planning team should number the site plan with all buildings and play equipment on the school grounds, recording the distances between features. The planning team will need to estimate the height of each of the buildings on the school grounds and record it on a separate set of notes, along with other characteristics of the building. Attachment A is an example of a building description sheet. It may be helpful to name areas or zones of the site if they do not already have a name. Zones can be named according to their use, such as "queuing area" or "passive play area." It is also important to document any significant topographical features, such as low spots, slopes, or ravines, because they will influence decisions on which shade strategies are most appropriate.

Because ultraviolet (UV) radiation can be reflected off ground and building surfaces, the planning team should make notes regarding the surfaces and finishes of each of the buildings and play areas on the school grounds.

Creating a Tree Inventory

The next task will require a degree of horticultural expertise. The planning team should inventory each tree and planted area on the school grounds, noting for each:

- Species.
- Estimated height.
- Trunk diameter.
- Condition (e.g., broken branches, dead limbs), paying particular attention to any that appear to be unhealthy.
- Estimated diameter of the tree's canopy, that is, the upper part which includes the branches and leaves.
- Density of the tree's canopy.

Trees should be numbered on the site plan and a separate set of notes should record the team's findings regarding each. Where densely planted areas of mixed species exist, notes should be made on which ones predominate. Attachment B is an example of a tree inventory data sheet.

Estimating the Height and Trunk and Canopy Diameters of a Tree

There are many ways to estimate the height and canopy diameter of a tree. Following is one method:

a. One member of the planning team first measures his or her own height in inches or feet.
b. The team member then stands next to the tree while another team member stands about 20 paces away.
c. With one eye closed, the second team member holds a pencil vertical at arm's length and covers part of the pencil so that the visible part is the same apparent length as the team member standing next to the tree.
d. Still keeping one eye closed, the second team member then moves the pencil up the tree and measures how many times taller the tree is than the team member standing next to it.
e. Multiply that number by the first team member's height and the result is a good estimate of the tree's height.
f. To estimate the canopy diameter, the second team member again closes one eye and holds the pencil at arm's length, covering part of

the pencil so that the visible part is the same apparent length as the tree height.

g. The pencil is then turned horizontal and, measuring at the canopy's widest point, used to determine how many times wider the canopy is than the tree's height.

To determine the diameter of a tree, simply measure the tree's circumference, usually at about 3 feet above the ground, and divide it by 3.14.

Describing a Tree's Canopy Density

The task of describing a tree's canopy density is somewhat subjective since there is no common metric. For the purposes of shade planning one could describe the density of a tree's canopy by rating it as "open," "moderate," or "dense." Standing beneath the tree and looking through its branches, if over 90% of the sky is blocked by the tree's canopy, it can be described as "dense." If between 50% and 90% of the sky is blocked by the canopy, it can be described as "moderate," and if less than 50% of the sky is blocked by the canopy, it can be described as "open." An open canopy provides little UV radiation protection.

Measuring Existing Shade

The final task of the shade audit is to estimate the amount of existing shade on the school grounds. Measurements should be taken of all shade, regardless of whether it is off-limits. There are two methods for measuring shade, one of which is highly technical and requires a working knowledge of both solar geometry and computer-assisted design software. The second method requires only that the planning team mark the shade patterns on the ground at the times of day that the school grounds are used. The ground can be marked with chalk, rope, or baking flour, then measured and marked to scale on the site plan. Measurements at several times during the day and throughout the school year will be neccesary to ensure that adequate shade is provided at the right time of day, throughout the year.

If the sky can be seen by those under a tree or structure, they are at risk for exposure to indirect UV radiation.

Considering Potential Shade Strategies

Having collected information regarding the activity patterns of the different users of the school grounds and the shade patterns cast by trees and buildings, it is now time for the planning team to assess their findings and make recommendations to the school community. The planning team might find that the school grounds provide adequate protection from both direct and indirect UV radiation; however, if not, the team will need to make recommendations for making more shade accessible to students, teachers, staff, and visitors. The team should first consider strategies that increase the amount of accessible shade at very low or no additional cost to the school. These might include revising school policies to allow access to off-limits shaded areas or relocating playground equipment or picnic tables to areas of the school grounds where shade already exists.

The planning team will also need to consider reflected UV radiation in their recommendations. These may include modifying ground and building surfaces to reduce their reflectivity. The planning team might determine that climbing vines would be the best solution for the indirect UV radiation reflected off a smooth wall or that artificial turf would be most appropriate to reduce the UV radiation reflected from a concrete playground.

The team should engage in a process to help them examine the cost effectiveness of strategies that could be employed as they are evaluating whether or not a particular strategy will accomplish the intended goal. More information about this is provided below.

The Shade Planning Matrix

The Shade Planning Matrix is a tool that can assist the planning team with comparing potential strategies for achieving their goals while examining and comparing the cost effectiveness of each of the strategies. The team's stated shade goals must be specific, both at this stage of planning and when it is time to present recommendations to the school community. The planning team should also clearly state any goals that are ancillary to providing shade, such as the construction of an outdoor classroom or the creation of a natural wildlife habitat. Matrices should be developed for each area that is being considered.

Information for completing the Shade Planning Matrix may come from a variety of sources. It could be necessary to request an informal quote from a contractor if the planning team is considering a solid-roof structure. Many vendors will provide prices over the internet if the team believes that a shade cloth structure would be an effective strategy. If a natural solution is being considered, the team will want to enlist the help of their United States Department of Agriculture County Extension Service agent, who can provide information on the most appropriate trees, shrubs, and vines for each geographical area, and the rates at which the vegetation is expected to grow. The Shade Planning Matrix is Attachment C.

Making Recommendations

When the team has considered potential strategies for achieving their shade goals and has arrived at a consensus on a set of recommendations, their final task is to formalize them in a report to the school community. Across schools and shade planning teams, considerable variability is likely in the report format. However, several components are essential:

The Rationale

Besides the most important reason, that shade provides protection from the harmful effects of solar UV radiation, the rationale should include any additional benefits that could be accrued through the strategies that the shade planning team has recommended. Those benefits might include the creation of an outdoor classroom and sheltered area for active play during inclement weather, provision of shade for athletic event spectators, or the creation of a wildlife habitat.

Statement of Goals

With as much specificity as possible, the statement of goals should include a physical description of the location, the amount of shade needed, and a description of the activities that occur. One example is the following:

The planning team has determined that there is a need to increase the amount of shade over the area of the playground bounded to the north by the south wall of the main building, to the east by the chain-link fence, to the south by the edge of the playground pavement, and to the west by the basketball courts. Based on patterns of use by the students, it is estimated that there is a need for a total of 2,500 square feet of shade. This section of the playground is home to the jungle gym and is popular for passive play as well. Because it provides an unobstructed view of the entire playground, this is where the playground monitors usually stand.

Strategies for Achieving the Goals

Strategies for achieving the goals could include moving playground equipment to a shaded area of the playground, revising school policy to make off-limit areas accessible, or building structures or planting trees to provide additional shade. The planning team should present their recommendations, but should also be prepared to discuss alternative plans.

If the team is recommending the creation of new shade, it should be prepared to discuss the performance characteristics of the materials providing shade, including:

- Where the tree(s) or shade structure will be located.
- The amount of shade that will be provided.
- Whether the need is for seasonal or year-round shade.
- The costs associated with providing the shade, including both initial and annual maintenance costs.
- The estimated lifespan of the building or tree(s) providing the shade.

Approaches for Achieving the Goals

The cost of providing shade can range from an afternoon of volunteer labor to the expense of building a large outdoor classroom with electricity and plumbing. The school district's budget for the project often cannot be known until the planning team presents their recommendations. For this reason, modifiable plans and alternate funding sources should be explored. While members of the planning team are completing the shade audit, other members can be exploring potential funding sources and volunteer resources. As the planning team presents their recommendations, they should also be prepared to present the options for advancing their plan. Options could include fund-raising efforts by the parent-teacher organization, donation of building materials by a local builder's supply store, or a tree planting project by a local Boy Scout troop.

Attachment A: Building Description

School: ______________ Date: ______________

Building Number	Name of Building	Height at Eaves	Height at Ridge	Wall Material	Wall Color

Attachment B: Tree Inventory

School: ______________ Date: ______________

Tree Number	Species	Height	Trunk Diameter	Canopy Diameter	Canopy Density	Age	Condition

Attachment C: Shade Planning Matrix

Area to be Addressed: __________

Current Status: ____________

Recommended Total _______
Square Footage of Shade:
Goal: ____________

Strategy 1:	**Initial Investment**	**Immediate Amount of Additional Shade**	**Estimated Annual Cost**	**Total Five-Year Cost**	**Total Shade at Five Years**	**Total Ten-Year Cost**	**Total Shade at Ten Years**	**Life Expectancy and Average Annual Cost**
Advantages:					**Disadvantages:**			
Strategy 2:	**Initial Investment**	**Immediate Amount of Additional Shade**	**Estimated Annual Cost**	**Total Five-Year Cost**	**Total Shade at Five Years**	**Total Ten-Year Cost**	**Total Shade at Ten Years**	**Life Expectancy and Average Annual Cost**
Advantages:					**Disadvantages:**			
Strategy 3:	**Initial Investment**	**Immediate Amount of Additional Shade**	**Estimated Annual Cost**	**Total Five-Year Cost**	**Total Shade at Five Years**	**Total Ten-Year Cost**	**Total Shade at Ten Years**	**Life Expectancy and Average Annual Cost**
Advantages:					**Disadvantages:**			
Strategy 4:	**Initial Investment**	**Immediate Amount of Additional Shade**	**Estimated Annual Cost**	**Total Five-Year Cost**	**Total Shade at Five Years**	**Total Ten-Year Cost**	**Total Shade at Ten Years**	**Life Expectancy and Average Annual Cost**
Advantages:					**Disadvantages:**			

End Notes

[1] MMWR 2002; 51(RR04):1-16. Available at http://www.cdc.gov/mmwr/review/mmwrhtm/rr5104a1.htm

[2] American Cancer Society. What Are The Key Statistics For Nonmelanoma Skin Cancer? Available at http://www.cancer

[3] American Cancer Society. What Are The Key Statistics For Melanoma Skin Cancer? Available at http://www.cancer

[4] American Academy of Dermatology. Skin Cancer. Available at http://www.aad.org/pamphlets/skincan.html

[5] Armstrong BK, Kricker A. How much melanoma is caused by sun exposure? *Melanoma Res*, 1993; 3: 395-401.

[6] Diffey, BL. Solar ultarviolet radiation effects on biological systems. *Physiology Medica; Biology* 1991; 36(3):299-328.

[7] United Nations Development Programme, Montreal protocol on substances that deplete the ozone layer. Available at http://www.undp.org/seed

[8] Williams ML, Pennella R. Melanoma, melanocytic nevi, and other melanoma risk factors in children. *J Pediatr* 1994; 124:833-45

[9] Moore LA. Ocular protection from solar ultraviolet radiation (UVR) in sport: factors to consider when prescribing. *The South African Optometrist* 2003; 62(2):72-79.

[10] Sliney, DH. Physical factors in cataractogenesis: ambient ultraviolet radiation and temperature. *Invest Ophthalmol Vis Sci* 1986; 27(5):781-790.

[11] Hall HI, Rogers JD. Sun protection behaviors among African Americans. *Ethnicity and Disease* 1999;9(1):126-31.

[12] Olson RL, Sayre RM, Everett M A. Effect of anatomic location and time on ultraviolet erythema. *Arch Dermatol* 1996; 93(2): 211-15.

[13] Diffey BL. Ultraviolet radiation and human health. *Clinics in Dermatology* 1998;16:83-9.

[14] Gartner LM, Greer FR. Prevention of rickets and vitamin D deficiency: new guidelines for vitamin D intake. *Pediatrics* 2003;111(4 Pt 1): 908-10.

[15] West SK, Duncan DD, Munoz B, Rubin GS, Fried LP, Bandeen-Roche K, et al. Sunlight exposure and risk of lens opacities in a population-based study: the Salisbury Eye Evaluation project. *JAMA* 1998;280:714-8.

[16] Rosmini F, Stazi MA, Milton RC, Sperduto RD. Pasquini P, Maraini G. A dose-response effect between a sunlight index and age-related cataracts. Italian-American Cataract Study Group.[comment]. *Annals of Epidemiology*. 4(4):266-70.

[17] Westerdahl J, Olsson H, Ingvar C. At what age do sunburn episodes play a crucial role for the development of malignant melanoma. Eur J Cancer 1994; 30A(11):1647-54.

[18] Zanetti R, Franceschi S, Rosso S, Colonna S, Bidoli, E. Cutaneous melanoma and sunburns in childhood in a southern European population. *Eur J Cancer* 1992;28A(6-7):1172-76.

[19] Elwood JM, Whitehead SM, Davison J, Stewart M, Galt M. Malignant melanoma in England: risks associated with naevi, freckles, social class, hair colour, and sunburn. *Int J Epidemiol* 1990;19(4):801-10.

[20] Gandini S, Sera F, Cattaruzza MS, et al. Meta-analysis of risk factors for cutaneous melanoma: II. Sun exposure. *Eur J Cancer* 2005;41:45-60.

In: Sun Safety for Schools and Youth
Editor: Jarrod C. Walton ISBN: 978-1-63463-067-2

Chapter 3

SUN SAFETY FOR AMERICA'S YOUTH TOOLKIT*

Centers for Disease Control and Prevention

1. ABOUT THE SUN SAFETY FOR AMERICA'S YOUTH TOOLKIT

Since 1998, the National Comprehensive Cancer Control Program (NCCCP) has provided funding and technical support to develop and implement comprehensive cancer control (CCC) plans to "reduce cancer incidence, morbidity, and mortality through prevention, early detection, treatment, rehabilitation and palliation."[1,2] Currently the Centers for Disease Control and Prevention (CDC) Division of Cancer Prevention and Control (DCPC) "funds CCC programs in all 50 states, the District of Columbia, 7 tribes and tribal organization and 7 U.S. territories."[3]

The CCC program in each state/tribe/territory/jurisdiction has a mandate to develop a plan that addresses a wide variety of cancer prevention and control priorities. This often includes skin cancer prevention. The Sun Safety for America's Youth Toolkit is designed as a resource for state/tribe/territory/ jurisdiction CCC programs interested in engaging schools and other education partners in sun safety efforts to reduce their state/tribe/territory/ jurisdiction's incidence of skin cancer. Since a majority of sun exposure occurs during

* This is an edited, reformatted and augmented version of a document issued by the Centers for Disease Control and Prevention, July 2009.

childhood and early adulthood[4] and key sun protective behaviors can most easily be established at this time, addressing sun safety for young people is an important cancer control objective.

There is a wide variety of sun safety programs, materials, and resources available to organizations interested in implementing sun safety efforts, many of which are described in this toolkit and the accompanying reference documents. This toolkit builds upon lessons learned from CDC's long history of sun safety and skin cancer prevention. In 2002, CDC released the *Guidelines for School Programs to Prevent Skin Cancer.*[5] The Guidelines provide resources and suggestions for schools to improve sun safety practices in seven major areas: policy, environmental change, education, family involvement, professional development, health services, and evaluation. To foster implementation of these guidelines, DCPC, in partnership with the Division of Adolescent and School Health (DASH), made funds available to states with Coordinated School Health Programs (CSHPs) to conduct pilot skin cancer prevention activities. In 2003, through the Skin Cancer Priority Supplement to PA03004—Improving the Health, Education, and Well-Being of Young People through Coordinated School Health Programs—three states (Colorado, Michigan, and North Carolina) were awarded funds to pilot activities to address the school skin cancer guidelines. From late 2003 through early 2007, the Department of Education in each of the three funded states received funds to implement their pilot sun safety initiatives. Each state was required to develop an annual work plan that would guide their efforts to address CDC's skin cancer guidelines and develop a partnership with their state CCC program.

This toolkit draws from these efforts and is designed to provide CCC programs with resources and information that will help them to understand the burden of skin cancer within their state/tribe/territory/jurisdiction, assess current state/ tribe/territory/jurisdiction-level sun safety interest and activity, engage in implementation of sun safety efforts with schools and key education partners, and evaluate their efforts. The toolkit consists of four key steps that will help CCC programs move through a logical process for engaging and implementing sun safety efforts for young people:

- Step I: Identify and Recruit Sun Safety Partners
- Step II: Assess and Understand Sun Safety Needs and Resources in Your State/Tribe/Territory/Jurisdiction
- Step III: Plan and Implement Sun Safety Activities
- Step IV: Evaluate Sun Safety Efforts

Step I describes the numerous organizations and individuals CCC programs may want to engage in sun safety planning and implementation. These partners represent both state/tribe/territory/jurisdiction and local organizations that can play an important role in reaching schools and young people to implement and enhance effective sun safety strategies.

Step II provides recommendations for understanding the current state skin cancer burden and how to utilize that information to inform the development and targeting of sun safety efforts. To understand the current level of sun safety activity within the state/tribe/territory/jurisdiction, recommendations and resources are provided for conducting a sun safety program and resource inventory at the state/tribe/territory/jurisdiction level. Resources are also provided to help your CCC program understand the current legal and/or policy issues related to sun safety and how sun safety may already be integrated into existing school resources and tools.

Step III outlines a process for conducting a Strengths, Weaknesses, Opportunities and Threats (SWOT) analysis related to implementation of sun safety activities. Recommendations and resources on selection of sun safety activities are provided as well as examples of activities implemented using the *CDC Guidelines for School Programs to Prevent Skin Cancer.*

Step IV highlights the importance of evaluation of state/tribe/territory/ jurisdiction sun safety efforts and offers some examples of how to evaluate sun safety efforts locally and at the state/tribe/territory/jurisdiction level. We also provide suggestions for modification of state surveillance systems.

Within each step, we provide examples from state sun safety efforts to help CCC programs understand how these recommendations, tools, and resources have been utilized by other states.

The toolkit also includes an extensive sun safety resource list, which highlights potential sun safety partners at the state/tribe/territory/jurisdiction and national levels, and other sun safety programs and materials that are currently available.

2. Why Is Sun Safety Important for Young People?

Skin cancer is the most common type of cancer and is thought to account for half of all cancers.[6,7] About one million cases of basal cell or squamous cell cancers, the two most common types of skin cancer, are diagnosed each year. Melanoma, the third most common type of skin cancer, [5] accounts for less than 5% of skin cancer cases but causes a majority of skin cancer deaths. [6,7]

Although children are not commonly diagnosed with skin cancer, it is during childhood that much of one's lifetime sun exposure occurs and when important protective behaviors can be established. Approximately 65%–90% of melanomas are caused by ultraviolet (UV) radiation,[5] and because a substantial percentage of lifetime sun exposure occurs before age 20,[4] UV radiation exposure during childhood and adolescence plays an important role in the development of skin cancer.[8] Persons with a history of more than one blistering sunburn during childhood or adolescence are at a greater risk for developing basal cell carcinoma[9] and are two times more likely to develop melanoma than those without such exposures.[5]

Why Is It Important to Work with Schools?

Sun exposure preventive behaviors can yield the most positive effects if they are initiated early and established as healthy and consistent patterns throughout life.[5] In 2003, the U.S. Community Preventive Services on Reducing Exposure to Ultraviolet Light recommended that primary schools implement educational and policy strategies to improve behaviors that reduce exposure to UV light by covering exposed skin and therefore preventing skin cancer.[10] Because much time during childhood and adolescence is spent at school, schools provide a favorable environment in which to teach and model healthy behaviors. There are approximately 50 million students attending more than 98,000 schools nationwide.[11]

Schools therefore provide the most far-reaching access to young people. Schools can play a critical role in educating young people about their health and ensuring that they have a healthy environment when they are at school and engaged in school activities. However, it is important to acknowledge that schools are faced with the challenge of maintaining high academic standards and addressing a wide variety of health priorities with limited time and resources.

Therefore, identifying opportunities to integrate sun safety into existing resources, activities, and curricula is critical to successful implementation and sustainability and to reducing burden on school partners.

In addition to schools, there are numerous other community organizations that provide services to young people and thus have an opportunity to educate them about the importance of sun safety. These organizations include parks and recreation departments, summer camps, museums, health education centers, and others.

Because of the important role these organizations and groups serve, they have been included as potential partners for any state/tribe/territory/jurisdiction sun safety effort.

3. STEP I: IDENTIFY AND RECRUIT SUN SAFETY PARTNERS

When preparing to engage in a sun safety effort, CCC programs can complement their own cancer control expertise by identifying and engaging additional partners who are knowledgeable and skilled in working with schools and young people. Such partnerships represent an opportunity for experts in cancer control and education to bring their respective areas of expertise together to identify strategies that can be implemented in a manner that reduces the burden on the educational system. These partners can facilitate sun safety activities in a number of ways, including

- building upon existing relationships to reduce potential barriers and reluctance by schools administrators and teachers to add sun safety to an already full agenda,
- serving as critical links to educate and improve school awareness and knowledge of the importance of sun safety,
- identifying opportunities to integrate sun safety into existing school programs and curriculum, and
- serving as sun safety advocates within their own organizations.

Develop Partnerships to Facilitate Sun Safety Planning and Implementation

In 2008, DCPC developed a *Partnership Tool Kit: Program Version*[12] that helps programs navigate the process of

- determining the need for a partnership,
- developing a partnership,

- evaluating a partnership, and
- sustaining a partnership.

This tool is recommended to CCC programs to help engage partners in skin cancer prevention efforts. Key aspects of this tool are included in this toolkit, but programs are encouraged to refer to the *Partnership Tool Kit: Program Version* for additional details and guidance.

When determining the need for a partnership, programs should consider the following questions:

- What specific outcomes or products does your program hope to achieve through partnerships?
- In what ways do you need partnerships to achieve the identified outcomes or products?
- How would partnerships provide additional expertise rather than duplicating expertise in your program?

Programs can then move toward developing a new partnership. Potential questions to consider at this stage include the following:

- What potential partners has your program identified?
- In what ways could nontraditional partners be helpful in a new partnership?
- What does your program aim to achieve by working with these potential partners?
- How will these potential partners complement and strengthen your program?
- What might be some potential drawbacks to working with these potential partners?
- How would these potential partners help your program better achieve your goals and objectives?
- What might your program and the potential partners gain through this partnership?
- What resources does your program have available to contribute to new partnerships?
- Is there an existing state-level school health coordinating committee?

Identify Other State/Tribe/Territory/Jurisdiction Partners to Engage in Sun Safety Planning

After assessing the need for additional partners and partnerships to promote a state/tribe/territory/ jurisdiction sun safety effort, CCC programs can identify a number of other state government agencies and programs that may serve as critical stakeholders and resources. The list below includes some examples of possible state-level partners that could be engaged in sun safety efforts. This list is not exhaustive, so each CCC program should identify other resources and partners specific to their state/tribe/territory/jurisdiction.

State Department of Education: The State Department of Education is an important stakeholder when addressing any issue that impacts young people. Twenty-two states and one tribal government are funded to build the capacity of their school systems through CDC's Coordinated School Health Program (CSHP).[13] The CSHP model consists of eight key components for a comprehensive health program: health education, physical education, health services, nutrition services, counseling and psychological services, healthy school environment, health promotion for staff, and family/community involvement. State health and education agencies are encouraged to develop an ongoing partnership to facilitate the implementation of effective policies and practices to promote the health and well-being of students and staff.

With or without funding for a CSHP, the State Department of Education represents a key partner in sun safety for young people and can provide valuable linkages, insight, and resources for engaging schools in sun safety. While health education classes are perhaps the most traditional mechanism for providing education on a particular topic, they are not the only avenues to be explored. Department experts or leaders in physical education, physical activity/wellness, school health services, and after-school activities are natural partners as they can incorporate sun safety into physical education classes and school sports activities. Sun safety can also be incorporated into a number of other academic areas, such as science and math (see the *Guidelines for School Programs to Prevent Skin Cancer* for additional information on incorporation of sun safety into various curricula); thus, it is important to try to identify partners beyond just the health education curriculum.

State Agency that Regulates Commercial Tanning Facilities: Every state has a state agency that is responsible for oversight, certification, and regulations related to indoor tanning/commercial tanning facilities (i.e., tanning beds). While not directly related to the schools, these organizations provide oversight to ensure that tanning facility staff are trained and that any state laws to protect minors from tanning are adhered to. Representatives from these agencies can be valuable partners for enforcement of existing state tanning laws or for development of such legislation if it does not already exist. A list of all state agencies responsible for commercial tanning facilities oversight can be found at http://www.tanningtraining.com/reginfo/state.html.

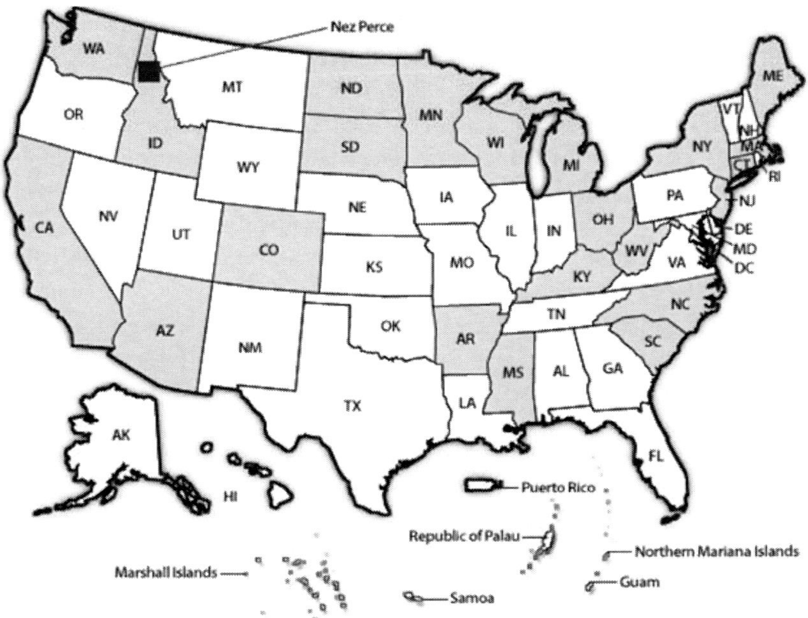

Note: State Education Agencies (SEA) that receive DASH funding are shaded. The tribal government from Nez Perce also receives CSHP funding. Source: CDC Coordinated School Health Program http://www.cdc.gov/healthyyouth/partners/funded/cshp.htm.

Figure 1. Coordinated School Health Programs (CSHP).

State Medical Associations: Clinical partners can play an important role in advocating for sun safe behaviors with adults and young people.*

* Links to non-Federal organizations found in this document are provided solely as a service to our users. These links do not constitute an endorsement of these organizations or their programs by CDC or the Federal government, and none should be inferred. CDC is not responsible for the content of the individual organization web pages found at these links.

- The National Association of School Nurses has affiliate school nurse organizations in 49 states (there is no affiliate in Hawaii) and the District of Columbia. State affiliate information can be found at http://www.nasn.org/Default.aspx?tabid=60.* School nurses play an important role in training teachers and students about practicing sun safe behavior and, in some cases, may have the responsibility of administering sunscreen to students.
- The American Academy of Dermatology (AAD) has affiliate State Dermatology Society organizations that can provide resources and support to sun safety efforts. AAD offers the Seal of Recognition Program and the Skin Cancer Awareness: Intervention Plan for Tomorrow (SCRIPT) Plan. The SCRIPT Plan includes a shade structure grant program, free skin cancer screenings, advocacy for federal and state legislation to regulate indoor tanning, paid and public service advertising, and sun safety resource materials. More information on AAD and its resources can be found at http://www.aad.org/index.html.*
- The American Academy of Pediatrics (AAP) has state chapters across the United States. AAP endorses a policy statement titled *Ultraviolet Light: A Hazard to Children*. Pediatricians can provide valuable information to children and parents on sun safety and can be a valuable advocate for passing state laws addressing skin cancer and skin cancer prevention. A list of state chapters can be found at http://www.aap.org/member/ chapters/chapters.htm.*

State Athletic and Coaching Associations: Young people are exposed to the sun during a variety of outdoor activities, including participation in school or community athletic activities. Including partners who represent state athletic and coaching associations provides a valuable resource for educating adults who oversee thousands of children during outdoor sports and athletic events about the importance of sun safety while on the field.

- The National Federation of State High School Associations includes member associations in each of the 50 states and the District of Columbia. A list of member associations and their contact information can be found at http://www.nfhs.org/stateassociations.aspx.*

* Links to non-Federal organizations found in this document are provided solely as a service to our users. These links do not constitute an endorsement of these organizations or their

Colleges and Universities: State colleges and universities often have a variety of experts, resources, and programs addressing sun safety, including

- Cooperative Extension Services,
- schools of medicine,
- schools of nursing, and
- schools of public health.

American School Health Association (ASHA): ASHA has state constituent chapters in 12 states and has passed a resolution supporting sun safety school policies and education to prevent skin cancer. A list of member associations can be found at http://www.ashaweb.org/i4a/pages/index.cfm?pageid=3317.*

Parent Teacher Association (PTA): The national PTA places an emphasis on healthy youth, and state PTA chapters can be valuable partners in implementing sun safety activities. State PTA chapters have access to local PTA chapters whose members can be educated to become suns safety advocates within their own school chapters. State PTAs can also pass resolutions and position statements in support of sun safety. State and local PTA chapters can be found at http://pta .org/jp find your pta .html.

Identify Local Partners to Engage in Sun Safety Planning

Depending on the sun safety approach and activities to be implemented, many CCC programs may also choose to engage local partners in their sun safety planning and activities. In many cases, local partners may be members or affiliates of state-level organizations that have already become engaged as sun safety partners. Local PTA chapters and individual health care providers are two examples of local organizations/members that may be closely affiliated with state-level organizations. There are a number of other local partners that can be engaged in sun safety planning and implementation.

Schools: Public, private, and alternative schools are perhaps the most obvious partners to engage in sun safety efforts, but also the most challenging. Learning how schools work is an important first step to working effectively with schools.[14] Because many policies impacting schools are implemented

programs by CDC or the Federal government, and none should be inferred. CDC is not responsible for the content of the individual organization web pages found at these links.

at the school level, it is often critical to work directly with schools and school administrators to integrate sun safety into school policies, curricula, and activities. Schools are faced with the task of addressing numerous student health issues while meeting or maintaining high academic standards. Gaining access to schools is often difficult and is most easily done by individuals and organizations that have preexisting relationships with schools and school administrators. While many schools are familiar with student health issues such as tobacco and drug use, obesity, physical activity, nutrition, and asthma, most schools are less familiar with the issue of sun safety. Engaging schools often requires time and resources to educate school decision makers on the importance of sun safety for their students and the approaches that a school can implement to protect students from the sun while in their care. Many schools have school health teams, and districts have school health councils that meet regularly to discuss school health problems and plans for improvement.

While the resources may not always be available, it is beneficial when even relatively small amounts of funding can be provided to schools interested in making improvements in sun safety policies, erecting or planting shade structures, or conducting education and awareness events and activities.

Local Education Agencies (LEAs): LEAs reside between individual schools and the Department of Education at the state level. LEAs are often considered school districts and provide administrative oversight to public schools in a particular geographic area. Like individual schools, LEAs can serve to provide leadership and guidance on school sun safety policies, shade planning, and curricula.

County or Area Parks and Recreation Organizations: While not directly related to schools, area parks and recreation organizations serve youth across the country, providing recreational sports activities, parks, and summer camps. Parks and recreation staff and the young people they oversee can benefit from educational and policy sun safety efforts. The National Recreation and Park Association was a sponsor of the Pool Cool sun safety effort aimed at improving sun safety behaviors of pool users. More information on Pool Cool can be found at http://www .poolcool .org/*

Health Education Centers: The National Association of Health Education Centers seeks to support and promote organizations that provide health education programs.

* Links to non-Federal organizations found in this document are provided solely as a service to our users. These links do not constitute an endorsement of these organizations or their programs by CDC or the Federal government, and none should be inferred. CDC is not responsible for the content of the individual organization web pages found at these links.

Thirty-eight member organizations can be found in 22 states and the District of Columbia. A list of health education centers can be found at http://www .nahec .org/documents/2007AnnualReport .pdf .*

LESSONS FROM THE FIELD

- Recognize that cancer control and education organizations have different structures, resources, and sometimes languages. It is important to take the time to learn what they are and how they can be used most effectively to promote sun safety efforts.
- Nurture the partnership through communication, development of goals, and setting timelines.
- Include partners who are familiar with education agencies at the local level so they can share what might and might not work with local sun safety efforts. These relationships can also help engage key school personnel who may serve as advocates or potential gatekeepers.
- Work with partners to create a plan of action, rather than approaching partners once a plan has been developed.
- Many potential partners and stakeholders are not knowledgeable about the issue of sun safety. There needs to be an effort to educate and improve awareness to recruit partners before many will be willing to engage in activities.
- Plan for sustainability from the beginning. Look closely at what kinds of activities and partnerships can help ensure financial and programmatic longevity.

Parent Teacher Organizations (PTOs): Many schools have parent groups that are not affiliated with the national PTA; these groups are often called PTOs. There is no national or state PTO, but each PTO is independently organized and operated.

Other Community-based Organizations: Many other types of organizations that serve young people can be included in sun safety planning and program implementation, including the following:

- YMCA: http://www .ymca .net/*
- YWCA: http://www .ywca .org/
- Boys/Girls Clubs: http://www .bgca .org/*
- Boy Scouts: http://www.scouting .org/*
- Girl Scouts: http://www.girlscouts .org/*
- Museums, especially those with outdoor activities: http://www .museumca.org/usa/states.html
- Zoos, aquariums, and amusement and water parks: http://www . themeparkcity.com/USA_index.htm*
- Minor league ball parks: http://www.littleballparks .com/*
- Public or community pools

4. Step II. Understand Sun Safety Needs and Resources in Your State/Tribe/ Territory/Jurisdiction

Once major partners are identified, CCC programs should undergo a process for understanding the sun safety needs, skin cancer burden, and existing sun safety resources within their state/tribe/territory/jurisdiction. Every state/tribe/territory/jurisdiction will have different types of resources already dedicated towards sun safety; thus, prior to implementing new interventions and activities, it is valuable to work with partners to conduct an assessment of what sun safety efforts are currently in place. This assessment can then be used to identify potential gaps in resources and sun safety needs and priorities.

Within Step II, we will provide recommendations on the following:

- assessing and understanding the skin cancer burden in your state/tribe/territory/jurisdiction,
- conducting a state/tribe/territory/jurisdiction–level sun safety inventory of existing programs and resources, and
- understanding your state/tribe/territory/jurisdiction's legal and/or policy issues related to sun safety.

* Links to non-Federal organizations found in this document are provided solely as a service to our users. These links do not constitute an endorsement of these organizations or their programs by CDC or the Federal government, and none should be inferred. CDC is not responsible for the content of the individual organization web pages found at these links.

Assess and Understand the Skin Cancer Burden in Your State/ Tribe/Territory/Jurisdiction

Assessing the burden of skin cancer in your state/tribe/territory /jurisdiction will allow your CCC program to prioritize strategies and interventions, and help focus efforts on particular programmatic and geographical areas with the greatest need. As most CCC programs are aware, there are a variety of national databases that provide state/tribe/ territory/ jurisdiction–specific data on the burden of skin cancer; however, tribe, territory, and jurisdiction data is not as easily available.

National Cancer Institute and centers for Disease Control and Prevention State Cancer Profiles: The objective of the State Cancer Profiles website is to provide a system to characterize the cancer burden in a standardized manner in order to motivate action, integrate surveillance into cancer control planning, characterize areas and demographic groups, and expose health disparities. The focus is on cancer sites for which there are evidence-based control interventions. Interactive graphics and maps provide visual support for deciding where to focus cancer control efforts. The State Cancer Profiles can be found at http://statecancerprofiles.cancer.gov/.

United States Cancer Statistics: This web-based report includes the official federal statistics on cancer incidence from registries that have high-quality data and cancer mortality statistics for each year and for 2001–2005 combined. It is produced by CDC and the National Cancer Institute (NCI), in collaboration with the North American Association of Central Cancer Registries (NAACCR).[1] The United States Cancer Statistics can be found at http://apps .nccd .cdc .gov/uscs/.

Data relating to the burden of skin cancer in your area can also be found in state, territory, and jurisdiction-based resources, including your state's cancer registry. The National Program of Cancer Registries (NCPR) and NCI's Surveillance, Epidemiology, and End Results (SEER) Program together fund 50 states, the District of Columbia, Puerto Rico, the U.S. Pacific Island Jurisdictions, and six metropolitan areas to conduct surveillance and develop and maintain a cancer registry for the area. Contact information for each state/ territory/jurisdiction cancer registry can be found at http://apps.nccd.cdc.gov/ cancercontacts/npcr/contacts.asp. Information on the NCPR can be found at http://www .cdc .gov/cancer/npcr/, and information on the SEER Program can be found at http://seer.cancer .gov/about/index .html.

Other tools are also available to help demonstrate the burden of skin cancer in your area.

Cancer Mortality Maps and Graphs: This site, sponsored by NCI, provides valuable information about cancer mortality in the United States during the time period 1950–1994, based on data obtained from the National Center for Health Statistics (NCHS). Cancer Mortality Maps and Graphs provides interactive maps, graphs, text, tables, and figures showing geographic patterns and time trends of cancer death rates for more than 40 cancers for the 50 states. This is found at http://www3 .cancer .gov/atlasplus/.

Skin cancer risk factor data is more difficult to obtain.

Youth Risk Behavior Survey (YRBS): The YRBS monitors priority health-risk behaviors among young people in grades 9-12. It has included the following questions regarding routine sunscreen use and routine practice of sun safety behaviors for the previous two iterations (2005 and 2007):

- When you are outside for more than 1 hour on a sunny day, how often do you wear sunscreen with an SPF of 15 or higher?
- When you are outside for more than 1 hour on a sunny day, how often do you do one or more of the following: stay in the shade, wear long pants, wear a long-sleeved shirt, or wear a hat that shades your face, ears, and neck?

In 2007, the YRBS was conducted in 44 states (although 5 states, Alabama, Colorado, Nebraska, New Jersey, and Oregon, did not obtain weighted data), the 22 districts, including the District of Columbia, and 5 territories and jurisdictions (Territory of Guam, Territory of American Samoa, Commonwealth of the Northern Marianas Islands, Republic of the Marshall Islands, and Republic of Palau). Information on the YRBS at the state and national level can be found at http://www.cdc.gov/HealthyYouth/yrbs/index .htm.

Several states, including Colorado, Florida, and New Mexico, have included skin cancer risk factor and sun safety related question in their Behavioral Risk Factor Surveillance Survey (BRFSS) during specific years. These questions can be found in Section 6 of this toolkit (Step IV).

Another data source that can be used to help your CCC program to prioritize strategies and target efforts on particular areas with the greatest need are school-based information systems. These systems can inform CCC programs about the location and demographic make-up of the schools in their area.

School District Demographic System (SDDS): The SDDS provides access to information about demographics, social characteristics, and economics of children and school districts from the U.S. Department of Education's National Center for Education Statistics (NCES). The SDDS enables users to directly access school district geographic and demographic data. This can be found at http:// nces .ed .gov/surveys/sdds/.

LESSONS FROM THE FIELD

- Understanding the skin cancer burden in your state can help your CCC program target limited resources toward the areas with greatest need. For example, if funds are available for mini-grants to schools, recruit schools from counties or geographic areas with the greatest prevalence of melanoma.
- If your state does not currently collect data on skin cancer or sun safety behaviors, adding questions to surveillance tools can help with understanding the state skin cancer burden and with evaluation of your sun safety efforts. These data can also be used to help demonstrate need, a critical requirement when identifying funding opportunities.

Conduct a Sun Safety Inventory: What Do We Already Know about the Available Resources around Sun Safety in our State/ Tribe/Territory/Jurisdiction?

Conducting a sun safety inventory will help your CCC program understand what types of activities and resources are currently available to schools and programs that serve young people. The partners identified in Step I are extremely valuable in completing this inventory as they will be able to provide insight and information about any existing sun safety efforts currently being implemented by their organizations and partners. Once an inventory is completed, the information can be analyzed and used to identify needs and/or gaps that your CCC program's sun safety efforts can work to address, thus ensuring that sun safety resources are used wisely and do not duplicate existing efforts.

Your inventory may include a number of different resources, several examples of which are provided below. In addition, a sample sun safety inventory tracking template is included as part of this toolkit.

Existing Sun Safety Programs in your State/tribe/territory/ Jurisdiction: There are a variety of well known sun safety programs and curricula used by schools and other community partners engaged in addressing sun safety for young people. When planning CCC sun safety activities, it is helpful to know if these programs and resources are already being used. Both the SunWise program and Sunny Days Healthy Ways are examples of programs that are recommended by the *Guide to Community Preventive Services*.[10]

SunWise: The U.S. Environmental Protection Agency's (EPA's) SunWise program is a free, school-based sun safety program that currently engages schools in all 50 states and the District of Columbia (http://www.epa .gov/sunwise/summary.html). The program is directed at educators in grades K-8 and includes a variety of materials and resources for the classroom, school, and community. Schools can register to be a SunWise school by completing a registration form online. As of 2008, 18,000 schools and more than one million students were engaged in SunWise (EPA, http://www.epa .gov/sunwise/evaluation.html). In spring 2009, CDC provided technical assistance to EPA as they began developing specific sun safety fact sheets for each state in the U.S.; the first fact sheets will be available soon at http://www .epa .gov/sunwise/.

As a part of your CCC program sun safety assessment, the SunWise program can provide your CCC program with a list of the schools that have registered with SunWise. While this does not ensure that a school is implementing all components of SunWise, it can serve as an indicator of school interest in sun safety and may help to target resources appropriately.

Sunny Days Healthy Ways: The Sunny Days Healthy Ways curriculum is designed for students and educators in grades K-8. The curriculum provides a wide variety of resources that can be tailored to the specific needs of schools and teachers. The curriculum also provides resources on incorporating sun safety into a variety of national and state health and science education standards (http://sdhw.info/standards/3 standards .asp).*

As a part of your CCC program sun safety assessment, the Sunny Days Healthy Ways program administrator, Klein Buendel, Inc., can provide you with a list of the schools that have purchased the Sunny Days Healthy Ways curriculum. As with SunWise, this does not ensure that a school is

* Links to non-Federal organizations found in this document are provided solely as a service to our users. These links do not constitute an endorsement of these organizations or their programs by CDC or the Federal government, and none should be inferred. CDC is not responsible for the content of the individual organization web pages found at these links.

implementing all components of Sunny Days Healthy Ways it can serve as an indicator of school interest in sun safety and may help to target resources appropriately.

Another popular sun safety campaign is the ***Slip, Slop, Slap*** sun safety media campaign and materials from Australia. Having launched Slip, Slop, Slap in 1981, Australia has one of the most well-established sun safety programs. This campaign encourages people to slip on a shirt, slop on some sunscreen, and slap on a hat. Most recently, the campaign has added seek shade and slide on some sunglasses.[15] This campaign has been used in several U.S. states and has been very successful in Australia. In addition to Slip, Slop, Slap, the Cancer Council Australia has a SunSmart Schools program that has engaged 2,500 schools and 3,500 daycare centers across the country.[16]

Other sun safety programs and resources that may be identified through an inventory include those presented in Table 1.

Organizations Already Engaged in Sun Safety: Step I of this toolkit provides examples of organizations that could be included as key sun safety partners. Many of the key organizations engaged in sun safety may have already been identified through this process. Additional organization may be identified by working with your state/tribe/territory/jurisdiction partners to brainstorm other potential organizational sun safety resources.

financial Resources for Sun Safety Activities: Identification of financial resources for implementation of sun safety efforts is often a critical component that determines whether schools and other organizations implement sun safety activities. A wide variety of free or inexpensive program materials are available to organizations interested in implementing sun safety activities, policies, and curricula. Many of these materials can be easily downloaded via the Internet. See the list of program resources included in this toolkit for links to many of these materials.

For projects around shade planning, a few grants and funding opportunities are available from national sun safety partners. The American Academy of Dermatology offers a small number of shade structure grants directly to schools each year, but these grants are highly competitive. Similarly, the SHADE Foundation of America offers occasional funding for the construction of shade structures at schools and play areas.

Table 1. Sun Safety and Skin Cancer Prevention Programs for Young People

Program	Sponsoring Agency	Website Information
Pool Cool	Rollins School of Public Health and the National Recreation and Park Association	http://www.poolcool.org/index.html*
Sun Safe for the Early Years and SunSafe in the Middle School Years	Norris Cotton Cancer Center	http://www.cancer.dartmouth.edu/melanoma/sunsafe_early.shtml* http://www.cancer.dartmouth.edu/melanoma/sunsafe_middle.shtml*
Block the Sun, Not the Fun	The Sun Safety Alliance	http://www.sunsafetyalliance.org/blockthesun.html*
Project S.A.F.E.T.Y (Sun Awareness For Educating Today's Youth)	M.D. Anderson Cancer Center	http://www.mdanderson.org/patient-and-cancer-information/cancer-information/cancer-education/prevention-programs/project-safety/*

Sun Safety in existing School resource materials and education Standards: In many states, the Department of Education has incorporated sun safety and skin cancer prevention into existing standard course of study materials, curriculum standards, and benchmarks. Sun safety has also been incorporated into many of the national health education standards and proficiency indicators (www.cdc.gov/healthyyouth/sher/standards/index.htm) and science education standards. An inventory should look to identify where sun safety is already included in school resources and standards and to identify potential opportunities for sun safety to be incorporated.

Human Resources: Because skin cancer affects millions of people across the United States, it is not difficult to find valuable advocates for skin cancer prevention and promotion of sun safety. These advocates can be found serving as school teachers, nurses and administrators, dermatologists, pediatricians, parents, grandparents, and skin cancer survivors. The identification and involvement of sun safety champions can be a valuable resource for implementation of sun safety activities. School health advocates often serve on district-level school health councils and school-level health teams.

Table 2. States with Laws Addressing Skin Cancer and Skin Cancer Prevention (enacted through March 2009)

State	Tanning Facilities	Prevention	School Health	Awareness	Health Education	Screening Reimbursement
Arizona	•	•	•			
Arkansas	•					
California	•	•				•
Connecticut	•					
Florida	•			•	•	
Georgia	•					
Indiana	•					
Kentucky	•	•	•			
Louisiana	•					
Maryland	•	•				
Massachusetts	•					
Michigan	•					
Minnesota	•					
Mississippi	•					
New Hampshire	•					
New Jersey	•					
New York	•	•	•	•	•	
North Carolina	•					
North Dakota	•					
Ohio	•					
Rhode Island	•	•				
Tennessee	•					
Texas	•					
Utah	•					
Virginia	•					
Wisconsin	•					
Total	**25**	**6**	**3**	**2**	**2**	**1**

Source: National Cancer Institute.[17]

Understand Your State/Tribe/Territory/Jurisdiction's Legal and/or Policy Issues Related to Sun Safety

There are a variety of legal and policy issues related to sun safety and skin cancer prevention that are important to understand and consider during the planning phase of any state sun safety effort.

Legislation related to Sun Safety: As of March 2009, 26 states had passed legislation regarding skin cancer or skin cancer prevention. This legislation is summarized in Table 2. Twenty-five states currently have legislation addressing access to and use of indoor tanning facilities. Between February and March 2009, three states (Montana, South Dakota, and Wyoming) failed to pass similar proposed legislation. Two states, Florida and New York, have passed laws promoting or requiring skin cancer education in schools.[17] A much smaller number of states have passed legislation regarding prevention, school health, skin cancer awareness, and skin cancer screening reimbursement.

Several resources are available to help CCC programs understand the current laws addressing skin cancer and skin cancer prevention.

- ***The National Cancer Institute's State Cancer Legislative Database Program*** provides a variety of resources on legislation related to cancer, including skin cancer and skin cancer prevention. It includes a searchable database to obtain information on skin cancer–related bills and resolutions: http://www .scld-nci.net/index.cfml.*
- ***The National Conference of State Legislatures*** provides a list of newly introduced and current legislation that addresses tanning restrictions for minors. A brief description of the restrictions is provided for each state along with links to each state statute: http://www.ncsl .org/programs/health/tanningrestrictions .htm

School Policies: In addition to legislative regulations related to sun safety, there is a variety of school policy issues that should be examined during a sun safety inventory. Many schools and/or local education agencies have established policies that impact sun safety, such as allowing hats and

* Links to non-Federal organizations found in this document are provided solely as a service to our users. These links do not constitute an endorsement of these organizations or their programs by CDC or the Federal government, and none should be inferred. CDC is not responsible for the content of the individual organization web pages found at these links.

sunglasses to be worn at school and use of sunscreen by students. Each CCC program should have an understanding of what policies currently exist within their state/tribe/jurisdiction/territory and where school policy decisions are made (i.e., at the state, local, or school level) to inform effective implementation of sun safe policies that reduce youth exposure to UV radiation. The National Association of State Boards of Education (NASBE) maintains the State School Healthy Policy Database, which "contains brief descriptions of laws, legal codes, rules, regulations, administrative orders, mandates, standards, resolutions, and other written means of exercising authority. While authoritative binding policies are the primary focus of the database, it also includes guidance documents and other non-binding materials that provide a more detailed picture of a state's school health policies and activities"[18] The database can be searched using state, topic, or key word searches.

LESSONS FROM THE FIELD

- Policies that impact schools are not always enacted through legislation at the state/jurisdiction/territory level. In many cases school districts, and in some cases individual schools, determine their own policies. It may be helpful to partner with individuals who work with schools to understand what local school policies are common in your state/tribe/jurisdiction/territory.
- Sun safety policy may not always be directly related to schools. Many states have policies that prohibit people under the age of 18 from using indoor tanning facilities. When assessing your state/tribe/jurisdiction/territory sun safety policy, do not limit your search to just school policies; expand it to include more broad sun safety policies.

5. STEP III: PLAN AND IMPLEMENT SUN SAFETY ACTIVITIES

Once you have identified partners and have a thorough understanding of the current sun safety resources and issues within your state/tribe/territory/ jurisdiction, you can move toward identification of sun safety priorities and strategies.

Conduct a SWOT Analysis

A Strengths, Weaknesses, Opportunities, and Threats (SWOT) analysis is a valuable process for most public health planning activities. The process helps an organization to identify strengths and weaknesses within an organization, and opportunities and threats outside of the organization that can help with planning and decision making. A detailed description of SWOT analysis is available at the University of Kansas Community Tool Box (http://ctb. ku.edu/tools/en/sub section main 1049 .htm*); a brief description of the brainstorming process is provided here.

Table 3. Sample Structure for Tracking SWOT Analysis Information

internal		external	
Strengths	**Weaknesses**	**opportunities**	**threats**

A SWOT analysis can help your CCC program explore options for new sun safety efforts and can help organize the information you have gathered through your identification of partners and sun safety inventory. The process should be conducted as a group meeting with key stakeholders and partners involved in the brainstorming process. Begin by using a table to outline your strengths, weaknesses, opportunities and threats (see Table 3).

After giving participants an opportunity to introduce themselves, explain the objectives for the SWOT analysis and the process that will be used. The SWOT process can be done in a large group or by breaking stakeholders out into smaller groups, but the groups should not exceed 10 people. Because a significant amount of work has already gone into the sun safety inventory, it may be helpful to provide SWOT analysis participants with a summary of what has already been found so that this may inform the brainstorming activity. Allow 20–30 minutes for the group or groups to brainstorm various strengths, weaknesses, opportunities and threats as they relate to the

* Links to non-Federal organizations found in this document are provided solely as a service to our users. These links do not constitute an endorsement of these organizations or their programs by CDC or the Federal government, and none should be inferred. CDC is not responsible for the content of the individual organization web pages found at these links.

implementation of a sun safety effort. Examples of possible internal and external factors are included below.

Internal Factors: Strengths and Weaknesses

- **Human resources:** CCC staff, state Cancer Control Consortium members, other state government agencies involved in sun safety, state sun safety partners, local sun safety partners
- **Physical resources:** CCC program offices, existing sun safety equipment or materials, partner offices in the communities or geographic areas where you may want to conduct sun safety activities
- **Financial:** CDC funding for sun safety activities, other state funding or resources that can be directed towards sun safety, funding from other sun safety or skin cancer prevention organizations
- **Activities and processes:** sun safety materials or resources managed by the CCC program or sun safety partners, existing surveillance systems
- **Past experiences:** the reputation and networks of the CCC program and key sun safety program partners (e.g., Department of Education) that will help facilitate new sun safety efforts, previous sun safety efforts implemented

External Factors: Opportunities and Threats

- **Future trends:** in cancer control (Is sun safety a priority given other cancer control needs?) and in student and youth education and safety (How can sun safety "compete for attention" with more well funded student health issues such as obesity and tobacco use?)
- **The economy:** local, state, or national (How will the current economy impact school resources and priorities for incorporating sun safety into current curriculum and activities?)
- **Funding sources:** state and national budget priorities, funds available from sun safety or skin cancer prevention organizations
- **Legislation and policy:** What skin cancer and skin cancer prevention legislation is already in place? How supportive has the state legislature been in addressing skin cancer and skin cancer prevention? What current school-level policies facilitate or inhibit sun safety practices?

- **Partners/partnerships:** What resources do partners have access to in order to facilitate implementation of sun safety activities? What partners are not yet involved but would be helpful?

Once the brainstorming time is over, a group leader can begin to ask each group to report on what they identified for each box (strengths, weaknesses, opportunities, and threats). A recorder should capture the contributions from each group, allowing for discussion while groups share their input or holding off on discussion until after all groups have contributed their thoughts. Continue gathering information from all groups until the table is complete.

What Do You Do with the SWOT Results?

Once the group has completed identifying strengths, weaknesses, opportunities, and threats, the group can do several things:

- develop consensus about the most important items in each category,
- relate the findings to the group's visions, mission, and goals for implementing a sun safety initiative for schools and youth, or
- begin to translate the findings into action plans and strategies for implementing sun safety efforts.

The SWOT analysis should help your CCC program and partners to "build on your strengths, minimize your weaknesses, seize opportunities, and counteract threats ."[19]

Select and Implement Sun Safety Activities

Building on what has been learned from sun safety partners, the sun safety inventory, and the SWOT analysis, a CCC program will be ready to explore what sun safety programs and activities should be implemented. There are a wide variety of school-based sun safety efforts, curricula, and activities that CCC programs can implement to keep young people sun safe. The U.S. Preventive Services Task Force has found that educational and policy interventions within primary schools have a positive impact on sun protective "covering up" behavior to reduce UV exposure. [10]

This includes wearing protective clothing, such as hats, shirts, or pants while outside. The evidence is limited as to the effectiveness of other skin cancer prevention interventions and activities, but there is still a great deal to be learned, so evaluation of sun safety efforts is of critical importance.

In 2002, CDC released the *Guidelines for School Programs to Prevent Skin Cancer*, which outlines seven guidelines schools can use to reduce the risk of skin cancer among students.[5] These guidelines, found at http://www .cdc .gov/ mmwr/PDF/rr/rr5104.pdf, provide resources and suggestions of how schools can work to improve sun safety practices in seven major areas:

1. Policy
2. Environmental change
3. Education
4. Family Involvement
5. Professional Development
6. Health Services
7. Evaluation

These guidelines serve as a natural starting point for any CCC program focusing on sun safety efforts aimed at impacting schools and young people. For those not familiar with the *Guidelines*, it is recommended that all guidelines be reviewed, and then programs select one or two to focus their efforts. When selecting guidelines to implement, it is important to work with your partners and utilize the lessons learned from the sun safety inventory and SWOT analysis to determine the strategies that are most appropriate.

In 2003, through the Skin Cancer Priority Supplement to PA03004, Improving the Health, Education, and Well-Being of Young People through Coordinated School Health Programs, three states (Colorado, Michigan, and North Carolina) were awarded funds to pilot activities to address the seven skin cancer guidelines. As a requirement of this funding, partnerships were established between each state's Department of Education and CCC program. Each state implemented activities using the guidance provided in the *Guidelines for School Programs to Prevent Skin Cancer*.[5] Examples of the types of activities implemented by these pilot states to address each of the seven guidelines are provided below.

LESSONS FROM THE FIELD

- Determine what teachers and schools are currently doing to address sun safety and how it may already be included in the curriculum. Where possible, look for opportunities to integrate sun safety into existing activities, resources, and curricula. Asking a school or partner to look for ways to incorporate sun safety in their existing activities will reduce any sense of burden that may accompany a request to add an entirely new topic to an already full list of responsibilities.
- School-related policy decisions in are often made at the local level rather than statewide, so rather than push for all schools in a state to change, advocates need to work within each school district or even within each school. Addressing these issues with each school can take more time and effort than would be required for a statewide policy.
- The school year ends in the summer, which is the prime time for people to think about sun safety issues. Motivating schools to think about sun safety in the fall and winter can be difficult because the topic may not seem as relevant at that time.
- CCC staff and partners may need to "sell" the idea of sun safety to schools and other organizations that serve young people. One valuable way of doing this is to identify ways to link sun safety with higher priority issues, such as physical activity, playground safety, and athletic/sports activities.

When selecting activities, it is important to consider the level of intervention at which your CCC program would like to intervene. Activities can be implemented at the local level (e.g., individual schools or LEAs, museums, YMCAs) or the state/tribe/territory/jurisdiction level (e.g., state PTA, legislature). Some guidelines are more easily applied at one level or another but which guidelines and activities are selected will be largely dependent on the type of activities your CCC program is interested in implementing. Each of the three pilot states funded under the Skin Cancer Priority Supplement to PA03004 utilized mini-grants to provide schools and partner organizations with funding to implement sun safety activities. The amount of funding varied but ranged from several hundred dollars to several thousand dollars. In one state, a large amount of funding was provided to the state PTA, which then distributed it in the form of smaller mini-grants to local PTA chapters interested in sun safety.

Providing a small amount of funding to schools and organizational partners served as an incentive for learning more about and implementing sun safety activities. An example of a mini-grant RFP is included as part of this toolkit.

The following are provided for each of the seven guidelines:

- a brief description of the guideline and why it is important to school-based skin cancer prevention efforts
- examples of program activities that have been implemented to address each of the guidelines.

The examples are largely drawn from states who implemented activities to address the *Guidelines* through a partnership between the State Department of Education and CCC program.

Please note that the evidence base of proven effective sun safety interventions is very limited. These activities are provided as examples of possible activities, but your CCC program should remain up to date on new evidence of effective sun safety interventions.

In addition to the information below, this toolkit includes a list of available resources to help your state CCC program address each of the seven guidelines.

Guideline 1: Policy – Establish Policies that Reduce Exposure to UV Radiation

Why Is Sun Safety Policy Important?

"An effectively crafted skin cancer prevention policy provides a framework for implementing the six other guidelines. The policy demonstrates institutional commitment and guides school and community groups in planning, implementing and evaluating skin cancer prevention activities… Although a comprehensive policy is preferable, more limited policies addressing certain aspects of skin cancer prevention also can be useful" (p. 7).[5]

Sample Activities

Local

- Offer mini-grants to schools and organizations to implement sun safety activities and require that each recipient include policy change in their efforts, in addition to any other activities.
- Provide sample sun safety policies to organizations and partners interested in implementing policies to remove the burden of developing new policies.
- Provide training and technical assistance to schools and other organizations on how to develop and implement sun safety policies. This can include training individuals who work with young people, such as teachers, school nurses, coaches, and PTA/PTSA groups.
- Disseminate resources such as *Fit, Healthy, and Ready to Learn* and CDC's *Guidelines for School Programs to Prevent Skin Cancer* to school boards and other decision making bodies. (Both of these documents are included as reference materials in this toolkit.)
- Help schools form school health teams and districts form school health councils to address health problems and promote health.

State/Tribe/Territory/Jurisdiction

- Work with state PTA partners to pass a sun safety resolution.
- Incorporate development of sun safety policy into state CCC plan.
- In states where current legislation does not exist, work with state agencies that regulate indoor tanning facilities to develop legislation to restrict tanning bed use by minors.

Guideline 2: Environmental Change – Provide and Maintain Physical and Social Environments that Support Sun Safety

Why Is Environmental Change Important?

"Policies can promote the provision of supportive resources for skin cancer prevention (e.g., shade, protective clothing and hats, sunscreen at a reduced price or free, and highly visible information and prompts for sun protection) in the physical and social environment. These policies help establish routine personal behaviors and social norms that promote skin cancer prevention in the context of organized group activities" (p. 9).[5]

Sample Activities

Local

- Conduct a shade audit using CDC's Shade Planning for America's Schools tools.
- Engage students in the research and design of shade structures that are appropriate for their school.
- Provide mini-grant funding to schools to build shade structures, plant trees, or purchase portable shade structures to be used at school events.
- Provide funding so that sunscreen can be purchased and provided to students and staff during school events (e.g., field trips, sports events, and field days). If necessary, obtain informed consent from parents so that students can use the sunscreen provided.
- Encourage school staff and students to wear sunglasses, sun safe hats, and shirts with sleeves when participating in outdoor activities.
- Produce and distribute sun safety fact sheets to parents, students, coaches, and teachers.
- Work with area parks, museums, health education centers, zoos, and community pools to provide shade structures for visitors.

State/Tribe/Territory/Jurisdiction

- Include questions on state school assessment tools to help schools identify ways to change the physical environment of their school to address sun safety. One example is the Healthy School Action Tool (HSAT) in Michigan. The SunSafe Colorado website also contains an assessment tool that can be used to assess the physical environment of schools.

Guideline 3: Education – Provide Health Education to Teach Students the Knowledge, Attitudes, and Behavioral Skills They Need to Prevent Skin Cancer

Why Is Sun Safety Education Important?

"Skin cancer prevention is likely to be most effective when it is taught as part of a comprehensive health education curriculum that focuses on understanding the relations between personal behavior and health (126) and that provides students with the knowledge and skills outlined by the National

Health Education Standards (112). … In addition to health classes, skin cancer prevention can also be integrated into other subject areas. …This type of integrated approach requires collaborative planning and curriculum development among teachers to optimize skin cancer prevention education and to ensure consistency of messages and practices" (p. 10).[5]

Sample Activities

Local

- Host an anti-tanning pre-prom fashion show that includes educational information about the dangers of tanning.
- Develop and disseminate anti-indoor tanning press kit to student newspapers and journalists.
- Partner with summer camps and parks and recreation organizations to implement a sun safety program for youth attending day camps and to train camp staff on staying sun safe.
- Provide UV detectors to students to increase awareness of sun exposure.
- Provide schools with sun safety information and resources, such as the Sunny Days Healthy Ways curriculum or EPA's SunWise program.

State/Tribe/Territory/Jurisdiction

- Integrate sun safety into existing teaching resources, including standard course of study guidance.
- Develop new sun safety resources or utilize some of the many that are currently available, including the SunSafe Colorado website (see Resource from the field box) or sun safety lessons in the Michigan Model for Comprehensive School Health Education.

RESOURCE FROM THE FIELD

The SunSafe Colorado website provides a wide variety of resources and information about sun safety for schools. The website was developed by their state partner Klein Buendel, Inc., who also developed the Sunny Days Healthy Ways curriculum. Klein Buendel has offered to work with states/tribes/territories/jurisdictions interested in modifying the SunSafe Colorado website to be specific to their state.

This would require a small amount of funding from your CCC program to make the necessary changes (e.g., logos, state data). If your state is interested in learning more about adapting the SunSafe Colorado website for your state/tribe/territory/ jurisdiction, please contact:

Mary Klein Buller, M.A. President, Klein Buendel, Inc.
1667 Cole Blvd., Suite 225
Golden, Colorado 80401 mbuller@kleinbuendel .com
303-565-4330 (phone)
303-565-4320 (fax)
www.kleinbuendel.com

Guideline 4: Family Involvement – Involve Family Members in Skin Cancer Prevention Efforts

Why Is Family Involvement in Sun Safety Important?

"Involving family members in skin cancer prevention efforts increases the likelihood that they will adopt and thus model healthful sun-protection behaviors of students (122). At a minimum, parents or guardians can be informed concerning school initiatives and policies and knowledgeable regarding how their cooperation is needed to ensure child health. Parents and guardians also can be encouraged to provide children with sun-protective clothing and sunglasses for outdoor activities. In addition, parents and guardians can serve as advocates for sun-protective policies and practices in schools" (p. 11).[5]

Sample Activities

Local

- Develop print or electronic resources specifically for educating parents about sun safety issues.
- Partner with state and/or local PTA groups to increase awareness of sun safety through presentations and, if possible, provide funds to PTA groups for sun safety activities.
- Include sun safety policies and information in student and parent hand-books and student planners.

- Distribute informed consent forms to parents asking permission for students to use sunscreen in school or at school activities and explaining the need for sun safety awareness.
- Distribute notes to parents about the importance of sun safety prior to field trips, field days, graduation ceremonies, and other outdoor events.
- Distribute sun safety information and sunscreen at community events, festivals, and celebrations that are held outdoors.

State/Tribe/Territory/Jurisdiction

- Partner with newspapers, parents' magazines, and organizational news-letters to publish and distribute articles and information on sun safety.
- Work with other state children's health organizations to identify other resources, publications, and meetings that could be used to educate families about sun safety (e.g., Cooperative Extension Children's Environmental Health Program).
- Partner with state and local media outlets to issue UV alerts.

Guideline 5: Professional Development-Include Skin Cancer Prevention Knowledge and Skills in Preservice and Inservice Education for School Administrators, Teachers, Physical Education Teachers and Coaches, School Nurses, and Others Who Work With Students

Why Are Professional Development Opportunities around Sun Safety Important?

"Appropriate and effective professional development efforts should be conducted for decision makers and care givers at all levels. Professional development activities, including certification programs and inservice education, are provided routinely for teachers and other school staff (e.g., coaches and school nurses). Skin cancer prevention can be integrated into those activities. All school staff should receive basic information concerning the importance of sun safety and key strategies for skin cancer prevention" (p. 11).[5]

Sample Activities

Local

- Train school staff and administrators on sun safety policy development and skin cancer prevention.
- Train camp counselors and others who work outside with youth during the summer on how to protect themselves and the youth they work with from sun exposure.
- Identify schools in regions with the highest melanoma rates and focus trainings in those communities first.

State/Tribe/Territory/Jurisdiction

- Collaborate with state sports/athletic associations to develop and/or provide training to coaches of outdoor sports teams.
- Provide training sessions on sun safety at other training or continuing education workshops for school staff, nurses, and teachers.

Guideline 6: Health Services – Complement and Support Skin Cancer Prevention Education and Sun Safety Environments and Policies with School Health Services

Why Is It Important to Engage Health Services in Sun Safety?

"School health services provide an opportunity for nurses, health educators, and school health resource specialists to promote and reinforce skin cancer prevention practices. Health professionals in the community, including pediatricians, primary care providers, nurses, pharmacists, and dermatologist are credible sources of information and guidance for skin cancer prevention. They can be advocates for skin cancer prevention policies, environmental changes, and programs, and support school programs through presentations, professional training, demonstrations, and classroom visits" (p.12).[5]

Sample Activities

Local

- Include school nurses in any trainings or workshops offered to teachers or other school staff.
- Provide mini-grant funding or other support to teen health centers to implement sun safety activities with teens and parents.

- Work with nurses and school administrators to discuss parental consent for sunscreen application at school.

State/Tribe/Territory/Jurisdiction

- Provide sun safety resources to your state Association of School Nurses and offer to attend and present at their meetings and conferences.

Guideline 7: Evaluation – Periodically Evaluate Whether Schools Are Implementing the Guidelines on Policies, Environmental Change, Education, Families, Professional Development, and Health Services

Why Is Evaluation of Sun Safety Activities Important?

Evaluation questions can be used "to determine whether their programs are consistent with CDC's *Guidelines for School Programs to Prevent Skin Cancer*. These questions can be used to (1) assess whether schools in their jurisdiction care providing effective education to prevent skin cancer and (2) identify schools that would benefit from additional training, resources, or technical assistance" (p.12).[5]

Sample Activities

Local

- Collect progress reports and final reports from mini-grant recipients to track their activities and progress.
- Track and document sun safety policies implemented by schools and other community partners.
- Conduct focus groups with teachers, principals, coaches, and school nurses to identify challenges and needs regarding sun safety activities.
- Conduct pre-post training evaluations to assess training events and changes in participants' knowledge, attitudes, and skills related to sun safety.
- Train mini-grant recipients on the importance of evaluation, evaluation expectations, and how to conduct an appropriate evaluation activity.

State/Tribe/Territory/Jurisdiction

- Add sun safety questions into state surveillance and data collection tools (e.g., BRFSS, YRBS).
- Identify state-specific surveillance tools that include sun safety items (e.g., NC Child Health Assessment and Monitoring Program, NC School Health Education Profiles, Michigan Healthy Schools Action Tools, Colo- rado Child Health Survey).

6. Step IV: Evaluate Sun Safety Efforts

Evaluation of your CCC sun safety effort is important for understanding and measuring the impact your program has on sun safety practices within your state and ultimately changes in state melanoma incidence. Evaluation is also important as a way to track progress toward meeting the goals and objectives in your state cancer plan. Evaluation results can be used to help identify and leverage additional sources of funding for your sun safety efforts and to inform program development and future sun safety program efforts.

The evaluation strategies your CCC program utilizes will need to be tailored to the unique goals and objectives of your cancer plan and to the types of sun safety strategies implemented. Evaluation planning should be conducted on an ongoing basis and should be initiated at the beginning of the program planning process to ensure that it is well integrated into your state efforts. There is a wide variety of evaluation resources available to your program. As an introduction to evaluation, please refer to CDC's *Framework for Program Evaluation in Public Health*.[20] Evaluation guidance and tools for schools are available from http://www.cdc.gov/healthyyouth/evaluation/ resources .htm. Several examples of local and state evaluation strategies are included under Guideline 7: Evaluation in the preceding section.

Inclusion of sun safety and skin cancer prevention questions in state surveillance tools and resources can yield important information regarding the current state of sun safety behaviors (as described in Step II under the heading Assess and Understand the Skin Cancer Burden in Your State/Tribe/Territory/ Jurisdiction). The BRFSS, YRBS, and other state surveillance systems can be utilized to assess both skin cancer burden and changes in behaviors.

LESSONS FROM THE FIELD

- Schools have limited resources for evaluating local sun safety efforts, so be specific about what evaluation data are required and be prepared to offer evaluation support.
- Include evaluation planning in your program planning process. It is helpful develop your evaluation plan while planning your program activities rather than waiting until activities are being implemented or have been completed.

Tables 4–7 present examples of questions that have been used on various national and state-based surveys to assess skin cancer risk factors and sun safety behaviors for both adults and children. Since the field of sun safety for young people is relatively new, there are more questions to assess adult sun safety behaviors than there are for young people. The YRBS has utilized several of the adult-focused questions when assessing sun safety behaviors of high school–aged young people. Table 8 presents questions regarding school-based sun safety education programs, including both student education and staff development questions. These questions could be added to state or local surveillance systems as one way to evaluate program progress.

Table 4. Skin Cancer Prevention/Sun Safety: Child-focused Questions

Question	Response Options	Citation
On average, when your child goes outside on a sunny summer day for more than an hour, how often does he/she use sunscreen or sun block?	a. Always b. Nearly always c. Sometimes d. Seldom e. Never	Colorado[21]
On a sunny summer day, on average how much time does your child spend outside in the sun between 11am and 3pm?	a. _ _ hours/ minutes b. Don't know/ not sure	Colorado[22]
When your child is outside for more than 15 minutes between 11am and 3pm on a sunny summer day, how often does he/she use sunscreen with an SPF of 15 or higher?	a. Always b. Nearly always c. Sometimes d. Seldom e. Never	Colorado[22] North Carolina 2005[23]

Table 4. (Continued)

Question	Response Options	Citation
On a sunny summer day, when your child is outside for more than 15 minutes between 11am and 3pm, how often does he/she stay in the shade?	a. Always b. Nearly always c. Sometimes d. Seldom e. Never	Colorado[22] North Carolina 2005[23]
On a sunny summer day, when your child is outside for more than 15 minutes between 11am and 3pm, how often does he/she wear clothes covering most of his/ her arms and legs?	a. Always b. Nearly always c. Sometimes d. Seldom e. Never	Colorado[22] North Carolina[23]
Thinking back over the past 12 months, tell me as best you can whether your child has had any sunburns during that time. By sunburn, I mean any reddening or burn of the skin that lasts until the next day.	a. Yes b. No c. Don't know/not sure	Colorado[22] North Carolina[23]
Do you think a tan makes a child look healthy?	a. Yes b. No c. Don't know/ not sure	Colorado[22]

Table 5. Skin Cancer Prevention/Sun Safety: Adult-focused Questions

Question	Response Options	Citation
When you go outside on a sunny summer day for more than an hour, how often do you use sunscreen or sun block?	a. Always b. Nearly always c. Sometimes d. Seldom e. Never	Honey[24] Colorado[25, 26] Kansas[27]
What is the SPF of the sunscreen you use mostoften?	a. _ _ Number b. Don't know/not sure	Colorado[25, 26]
When you go outside on a sunny summer day for more than an hour, how often do you stay in the shade?	a. Always b. Nearly always c. Sometimes d. Seldom e. Never	Colorado[25, 26] Kansas[27]

Question	Response Options	Citation
When you go outside on a sunny day for more than an hour, how often do you wear a wide-brimmed hat or any other hat that shades your face, ears, and neck from the sun?	a. Always b. Nearly always c. Sometimes d. Seldom e. Never	Honey[24] Colorado[25, 26] Kansas[27]
When you go outside on a sunny summer day for more than an hour, how often do you wear long-sleeved shirts?	a. Always b. Nearly always c. Sometimes d. Seldom e. Never	Colorado[25, 26] Kansas[27]
When you are tanning, either outside or on an indoor tanning bed, what products do you usually apply to your skin?	a. Tan enhancer b. Sunscreen with SPF less than 15 c. Sunscreen with SPF 15 or higher d. I do not use any skin products e. I do not purposely tan in direct sunlight or use a tanning bed f. Other	Florida[28]
When you are outside in direct sunlight for the purpose of tanning, do you reapply sunscreen?	a. Yes b. No c. I do not purposely tan in direct sunlight d. Don't know/not sure	Florida[28]
Have you used a tanning bed or sun lamp in the last 12 months?	a. Yes b. No	Kansas[27]
Has a doctor, nurse, or other health professional ever spoken with you about taking protective measures against skin cancer? Protective measures include use of sunscreen, protective clothing, and avoiding exposure to sunlamps or tanning beds.	a. Yes, within the past year(any time less than 12 months ago) b. Yes, within the past 2 years(1 year but less than 2 years ago) c. Yes, within the past 3 years(2 years but less than 3 years ago) d. Yes, within the past 5 years(2 years but less than 5 years ago)	Kansas[29]

Table 5. (Continued)

Question	Response Options	Citation
	e. Yes, 5 or more years ago f. No	
Including any time that even a small part of your skin was red for more than 12 hours, have you had a sunburn within the past 12 months?	a. Yes b. No	Kansas[30]
Including times when even a small part of your skin was red for more than 12 hours, how many sunburns have you had within the past 12 months?	a. One b. Two c. Three d. Four e. Five f. Six or more	Kansas[30]

Table 6. Skin Cancer Risk Factors: Adult-focused Questions

Question	Response Options	Citations
Have you had a sunburn within the past 12 months?	a. Yes b. No c. Don't know/not sure	Honey[24] Colorado[25, 26] Florida[31]
Including times when even a small part of your skin was red for more than 12 hours, how many sunburns have you had within the past 12 months?	a. One b. Two c. Three d. Four e. Five f. Six or more g. Don't know/not sure	Colorado[25, 26] Florida[31]

Table 7. Sun Safety Perception: Adult-focused Question

Question	Response Options	Citation
Suppose that after several months of not being out in the sun, you went out in the sun without a hat, sunscreen, or protective clothing for an hour. Would you sunburn, darken without sunburn, or not have anything happen?	a. Sunburn b. Darken without sunburn c. Not have anything happen	Honey[24]

Table 8. School-based Education/Program Implementation

Question	Response Options	Citation
Now I am going to read a list of health topics. For each one, please tell me if you support school children receiving age-appropriate education about it in school.	a. Dental and oral health b. Nutrition and dietary behavior c. Human sexuality d. Sexually transmitted disease prevention e. Emotional and mental health f. Suicide prevention g. Tobacco use prevention h. Alcohol and other drug use prevention i. Violence prevention j. Sun safety	Colorado[22]
Does your school have a policy establishing sun safety guidelines for any of the following areas?	a. Encourage or allow students to apply lip balm and/or sunscreen b. New construction/ renovation projects include a plan for shade areas c. Promote or require the use of protective clothing outside (e.g., hats, sunglasses) d. Sun safety staff development opportunities for teachers e. Sun safety education for students f. Other areas	North Carolina[32]
During this school year, have teachers in this school tried to increase student knowledge on each of the following topics in a required health education course in any of grades 6 through 12? ***- Sun safety or skin cancer prevention***	a. Yes b. No	CDC[33]

Table 8. (Continued)

Question	Response Options	Citation
During this school year, did teachers in this school teach each of the following physical activity topics in a required health education course for students in any of grades 6 through 12? ***- Weather-related safety (e.g., avoiding heat stroke, hypothermia, and sunburn while physically active)***	a. Yes b. No	CDC[33]
During the past 2 years, did you receive staff development (such as workshops, conferences, continuing education, or any other kind of inservice) on each of the following health education topics? ***- Sun safety or skin cancer prevention***	a. Yes b. No	CDC[33]
Would you like to receive staff development on each of these health education topics? ***-Sun safety or skin cancer prevention***	a. Yes b. No	CDC[33]

CONCLUSION

Protecting young people from UV exposure and teaching them how to practice lifelong sun safety behaviors is critical to reducing the rates of skin cancer in our country. As we have demonstrated, there is an abundance of informational material available to support programs and schools interested in engaging in sun safety activities. This toolkit brings together many of these resources into one package so that your program may develop and select sun safety strategies to address the needs of your state and program.

REFERENCES

[1] Centers for Disease Control and Prevention (CDC). (2009). *Coordinated School Health Program.* Retrieved May 4, 2009, from http://www.cdc .gov/healthyyouth/ partners/funded/cshp_map .htm.

[2] Centers for Disease Control and Prevention (CDC). (2009). *National Comprehensive Cancer Control Program (NCCCP).* Retrieved May 4, 2009, from http://www .cdc .gov/cancer/ncccp/about .htm.

[3] Centers for Disease Control and Prevention (CDC). (2008/2009). *Comprehensive Cancer Control Program.* Retrieved May 4, 2009, from http://www .cdc .gov/cancer/ ncccp/cccpdf/0809_ncccp_fs .pdf.

[4] Godar, D. E. (2001). UV doses of American children and adolescents . *Photochemistry and Photobiology, 74*(6), 787–793.

[5] Centers for Disease Control and Prevention (CDC). (2002). Guidelines for school programs to prevent skin cancer. *Morbidity and Mortality Weekly Report, 51*(No.RR-4), 1-20.

[6] American Cancer Society (ACS). (2008). *Detailed guide: Skin cancer—basal and squamous cell. What are the key statistics about squamous and basal cell skin cancer?* Retrieved May 25, 2008, from http://www .cancer.org/docroot/CRI/content/CRI_2_2_1X_How_many_people_ get_nonmelanoma_skin_cancer_51. asp?sitearea= .

[7] American Cancer Society (ACS). (2008) . *Detailed guide: Skin cancer—melanoma. What are the key statistics about melanoma?* Retrieved May 25, 2008, from http:// www .cancer .org/docroot/CRI/content/CRI 2 4 1X What are the key statistics for_melanoma_50 .asp?sitearea= .

[8] Gilchrest, B. A., Eller, M. S., Geller, A. C. & Yaar, M. (1999). The pathogenesis of melanoma induced by ultraviolet radiation. *New England Journal of Medicine, 340,* 1341–1348.

[9] Kricker, A., Armstrong, B. K., English, D. R., et al. (1995). Does intermittent sun exposure cause basal cell carcinoma? A case-control study in Western Australia. *International Journal of Cancer, 60*, 489–494.

[10] Centers for Disease Control and Prevention (CDC). (2003). Preventing skin cancer: Findings of the Task Force on Community Preventive Services on reducing exposure to ultraviolet light and counseling to prevent skin cancer, recommendations and rationale of the U.S. Preventive Services Task Force. *Morbidity and Mortality Weekly Report, 52*(No. RR-15), 1–18.

[11] U.S. Department of Education. (2008). *Mapping America's Educational Progress 2008.*Retrieved June 21, 2008, from http://www.ed.gov/nclb/ accountability/results/progress/nation .html .
[12] Soloe, C. (2007). *Developing, maintaining, and sustaining partnerships* . Final report prepared for CDC Division of Cancer Prevention and Control.
[13] Centers for Disease Control and Prevention (CDC). (2008). *Healthy youth! Coordinated school health program.* Retrieved June 21, 2008, from http://www .cdc . gov/healthyyouth/CSHP .
[14] Bogden, J. F. (2003). *How schools work and how to work with schools: A primer for professionals who serve children and youth* . Alexandria, VA: National Association of State Boards of Education .
[15] Cancer Council Australia. (2009). *Slip, slop, slap.* Retrieved June 1, 2009, from http://www.cancer.org.au/cancersmartlifestyle/SunSmart/ Campaignsandevents/ SlipSlopSlap.htm .
[16] Cancer Council Australia . (2009). *Sun smart schools* . Retrieved June 1, 2009, from http://www.cancer.org.au/cancersmartlifestyle/ SunSmart/ SunSmartschools.htm .
[17] National Cancer Institute. (2005). *State cancer legislative database program.* Bethesda, MD: National Cancer Institute.
[18] National Association of State Boards of Education (2009). *State school health policy database.* Retrieved June 5, 2009, from http://nasbe.org/ index.php/shs/health- policies-database.
[19] The Community Toolbox. (2009). *SWOT analysis: Strengths, weaknesses, opportunities and threats.* Retrieved May 28, 2009, from http://ctb.ku.edu/en/ tablecontents/sub_section_main_1049.htm.
[20] Centers for Disease Control and Prevention (CDC). (1999). Framework for program evaluation in public health. *Morbidity and Mortality Weekly Report, 48*(No . RR-11) .
[21] Colorado Department of Public Health and Environment. (2006). *2002 Colorado behavioral risk factor surveillance system questionnaire.* Retrieved May 26, 2009, from http://www.cdphe.state.co.us/hs/brfss/ FinalCO02 .pdf .
[22] Colorado Department of Public Health and Environment. (2005). *2005 Colorado child health survey questionnaire.* Retrieved May 26, 2009, from http://www.cdphe. state.co.us/hs/mchdata/chs2005 .pdf.
[23] North Carolina State Center for Health Statistics. (2005). *2005 North Carolina CHAMP child health assessment and monitoring program*

survey. Retrieved May 26, 2009, from http://www.schs.state.nc.us/SCHS/champ/pdf/CHAMPQ05 .pdf.

End Note

[1] U.S. Cancer Statistics Working Group. United States Cancer Statistics: 1999–2005 Incidence and Mortality Web-based Report. Atlanta: U.S. Department of Health and Human Services, Centers for Disease Control and Prevention and National Cancer Institute; 2009. Available at: www.cdc.gov/uscs.

INDEX

A

access, 61, 101, 110, 116, 117, 121, 127, 131
accountability, 18, 150
acid, 10, 28
acne, 28
acoustics, 61
actinic keratosis, 54
administrators, viii, 14, 16, 25, 26, 44, 67, 92, 111, 117, 125, 140, 141
adolescents, vii, viii, 1, 3, 6, 11, 12, 22, 23, 38, 47, 53, 149
adulthood, ix, 6, 33, 108
adults, 6, 11, 17, 20, 38, 46, 53, 114, 115, 143
adverse effects, 10
adverse event, 10
advocacy, 16, 56, 115
aesthetics, 46, 63
African Americans, 38, 106
age, vii, viii, 1, 2, 3, 5, 7, 11, 12, 14, 31, 32, 54, 57, 74, 79, 93, 94, 106, 110, 128, 143, 147
agencies, viii, 2, 13, 25, 26, 29, 113, 114, 118, 127, 130, 135
AIDS, 31
allergens, 10
allergic reaction, 10, 63
ambient air, 76
American Samoa, 121
anatomic site, 34
architects, 17, 68, 72, 92
assessment, 35, 91, 119, 123, 136, 150
assessment tools, 136
asthma, 117
athletes, 55
atmosphere, 48, 50, 88
attitudes, viii, 12, 14, 18, 20, 22, 26, 37, 38, 43, 141
audit(s), 48, 66, 68, 70, 71, 72, 90, 91, 97, 100, 103, 136
authority, 128
avoidance, 8, 53
awareness, 20, 40, 55, 57, 111, 117, 118, 127, 137, 138, 139

B

background information, 56, 68
barriers, 94, 95, 96, 97, 111
basal cell carcinoma, 3, 5, 6, 9, 33, 54, 110, 149
base, 134
behavioral change, 13, 21
behaviors, ix, 2, 9, 11, 12, 13, 14, 19, 20, 22, 23, 24, 25, 37, 38, 55, 57, 80, 97, 106, 108, 110, 114, 117, 121, 122, 135, 138, 142, 143, 148
Belgium, 35

benchmarks, 125
beneficial effect, 52
benefits, 35, 64, 66, 73, 102
biological systems, 32, 106
birds, 60, 64, 66, 79
blood, 52
blood vessels, 52
board members, 47, 75
bones, 12
brainstorming, 129, 131
building code, 59, 72
burn, 5, 51, 62, 144
businesses, 59, 69, 77, 98

C

cables, 75
calcium, 39, 53
cancer control, ix, 107, 108, 111, 118, 120, 130
cancer death, 4, 44, 110, 121
Cancer Prevention and Control, ix, 29, 43, 107, 150
cancer screening, 80, 127
carbon, 50
carbon tetrachloride, 50
carcinoma, 3, 4, 9, 33
cardiovascular disease, 39
caregivers, 18, 24, 57, 80
case study(s), 74
cataract, 32
CCC, ix, x, xi, 107, 108, 109, 111, 112, 113, 116, 119, 120, 121, 122, 123, 127, 128, 129, 130, 131, 132, 133, 134, 135, 138, 142
CDC, viii, ix, xi, 2, 3, 25, 29, 31, 38, 43, 46, 55, 58, 107, 108, 109, 113, 114, 116, 117, 119, 120, 123, 127, 129, 130, 132, 135, 136, 141, 142, 147, 148, 149, 150
Census, 74, 77
Centers for Disease Control and Prevention, v, viii, ix, 1, 43, 55, 58, 107, 149, 150, 151
certification, 24, 113, 139
challenges, 41, 141
chemical(s), 9, 10, 28, 50
child development, 73
childhood, vii, ix, 1, 2, 6, 16, 27, 31, 33, 38, 46, 54, 55, 106, 108, 110
children, vii, viii, 1, 3, 10, 11, 12, 15, 17, 18, 19, 22, 23, 24, 25, 33, 35, 36, 37, 38, 40, 41, 47, 53, 55, 56, 57, 62, 75, 77, 78, 79, 80, 81, 82, 106, 110, 115, 122, 138, 139, 143, 147, 149, 150
chloroform, 50
chronic diseases, 11, 46
circulation, 76
cities, 65, 73
class period, 57
classes, 17, 21, 45, 75, 78, 113, 137
classroom, 22, 25, 45, 56, 57, 58, 59, 60, 61, 64, 65, 80, 94, 95, 96, 101, 102, 103, 123, 140
climate(s), 21, 23
clothing, 3, 5, 8, 10, 11, 12, 15, 16, 17, 19, 24, 27, 28, 35, 36, 131, 135, 138, 145, 146, 147
coaches, viii, 14, 16, 18, 24, 41, 44, 67, 69, 135, 136, 139, 140, 141
collaboration, viii, 2, 56, 73, 74, 80, 120
colleges, 116
color, 6, 8, 9, 50, 52, 54
colorectal cancer, 32
commercial, 57, 113
communication, 118
community(s), viii, ix, 3, 12, 13, 15, 16, 17, 19, 22, 23, 25, 26, 31, 39, 40, 41, 43, 44, 46, 52, 56, 57, 64, 65, 66, 72, 80, 82, 110, 113, 115, 119, 123, 130, 134, 136, 139, 140, 141
community service, 72
compaction, 63
complement, 23, 111, 112
computer, 22, 40, 90, 100
computer software, 90
computer technology, 40
conference, 31
consensus, 3, 67, 102, 131
constituents, 2, 15, 16

construction, 8, 19, 59, 68, 75, 76, 77, 78, 101, 124, 147
cooperation, 16, 24, 138
Cooperative State Research, Education, and Extension Service, 65
correlation, 34
cost, 56, 59, 60, 63, 75, 76, 78, 81, 82, 101, 103
cost benefit analysis, 76
cost effectiveness, 101
cotton, 8
counseling, 8, 13, 25, 41, 113, 149
covering, 99, 110, 131, 144
CST, 49
cues, 20
culture, 65
curricula, 22, 23, 24, 26, 46, 55, 56, 110, 113, 117, 123, 124, 131, 133
curriculum, 20, 21, 40, 56, 57, 80, 81, 82, 111, 113, 123, 125, 130, 133, 136, 137
curriculum development, 21, 137

D

danger, 62
data collection, 68, 142
database, 127, 128, 150
DCPC, ix, 107, 108, 111
death rate, 4
deaths, vii, 1, 3, 4
decision makers, 24, 117, 139
decision-making process, 72
demographic data, 122
demonstrations, 25, 140
Department of Agriculture, 63, 65, 102
Department of Education, x, 108, 113, 117, 122, 125, 130, 132, 134, 150
Department of Health and Human Services, 31, 151
dermatologist, 19, 140
dermatology, viii, 2
designers, 78
detection, ix, 4, 31, 56, 80, 107
diamonds, 69
diet, 12
dilation, 52
diseases, 26
disorder, 12
distribution, 31, 93
District of Columbia, ix, 57, 107, 115, 118, 120, 121, 123
diversity, 73
DNA, 4
doctors, 4
dose-response relationship, 54
drainage, 59, 63
drawing, 68, 75, 90, 92
drying, 10

E

economics, 122
ecosystem, 65
educational materials, 24
educational programs, vii, viii, 2, 16, 22, 23, 80
educational system, 111
educators, 16, 20, 25, 55, 64, 123, 140
electricity, 103
electromagnetic, 48
elementary school, 22, 40, 56, 57, 60, 74, 75, 76, 77, 78, 79
emergency, 20
enforcement, 114
England, 33, 35, 106
environment(s), viii, 2, 12, 13, 14, 15, 17, 20, 23, 39, 44, 46, 55, 64, 73, 78, 80, 81, 110, 113, 136
environmental change, vii, viii, ix, 2, 13, 14, 25, 26, 44, 108, 140
environmental organizations, 72
Environmental Protection Agency (EPA), 22, 30, 40, 51, 52, 55, 56, 57, 66, 74, 79, 80, 81, 82, 83, 123, 137
epidemiologic, 7, 32, 35, 36
epidemiologic studies, 32
epidemiology, 4, 31, 34
equipment, 69, 76, 98, 101, 103, 130
EST, 49
evidence, 3, 4, 7, 54, 120, 131, 134

examinations, 25
exercise, 21, 28, 58
expertise, 67, 68, 69, 78, 90, 99, 111, 112

F

families, viii, 2, 13, 14, 16, 19, 20, 23, 26, 139
family history, 7
family members, viii, 14, 23, 43, 138
family support, 23
farms, 3
federal government, 15, 45, 55
federal regulations, 9
fiber(s), 8, 53
fights, 77
financial, 17, 65, 72, 118, 124
financial resources, 124
fish, 12
flexibility, 58, 59, 81
flour, 70, 100
focus groups, 141
forest resources, 65
formation, 32
formula, 12, 53
framing, 60, 79
France, 27, 32, 34, 35
fruits, 63
funding, ix, 18, 19, 24, 72, 103, 107, 113, 114, 117, 122, 124, 130, 132, 133, 136, 138, 140, 142
funds, ix, 75, 77, 82, 107, 108, 122, 130, 132, 138

G

geometry, 48, 84, 90, 91, 100
Georgia, 41, 126
Germany, 35
grades, 23, 56, 57, 121, 123, 147, 148
grants, 72, 81, 82, 122, 124, 133, 135
grass, 46, 50
greening, 73
group activities, 19, 20, 135
growth, 71
guidance, 25, 112, 117, 128, 132, 137, 140, 142
guidelines, vii, viii, ix, 2, 3, 8, 10, 13, 14, 15, 26, 31, 36, 43, 74, 77, 106, 108, 132, 133, 134, 147
Gulf of Mexico, 77

H

habitat(s), 64, 101, 102
hair, 6, 52, 106
harmful effects, 63, 102
Hawaii, 40, 41, 115
HE, 40
head lice, 18
health care, 116
health education, 2, 13, 14, 18, 20, 21, 22, 23, 31, 39, 57, 80, 111, 113, 117, 125, 136, 147, 148
health information, 33
health problems, 117, 135
health promotion, 13, 113
health risks, 55, 57
health services, viii, ix, 2, 13, 14, 25, 26, 44, 108, 113, 140
heat stroke, 148
height, 70, 88, 98, 99, 100
hemisphere, 49, 83, 86, 87, 88
high school, 16, 23, 38, 143
high winds, 59
higher education, 3, 13
high-risk populations, 55
Hispanics, 6
history, vii, ix, 1, 6, 7, 21, 37, 108, 110
homes, 69, 98
human, 17, 55, 106
human health, 55, 106
human resources, 17
hurricanes, 76, 78
hygiene, 20
hypothermia, 148

I

ideal, 18
identification, 125, 128, 129
images, 23, 65
immune system, 5
improvements, 22, 24, 79, 94, 96, 117
incidence, ix, 2, 4, 5, 6, 7, 9, 31, 32, 34, 37, 44, 46, 90, 107, 120, 142
individuals, x, 34, 66, 67, 97, 109, 117, 128, 135
industry, 9
infants, 12, 53, 55
informed consent, 136, 139
ingredients, 10, 25, 28
injury(s), 37, 46, 52
institutions, 3, 13, 17
instructional materials, 65
integration, 26
integrity, 62
intervention, 57, 133
investment, 39
issues, 47, 55, 68, 79, 93, 117, 128, 130, 133, 138

J

journalists, 137
jurisdiction(s), ix, x, xi, 25, 107, 108, 109, 111, 113, 119, 120, 124, 128, 133, 135, 136, 137, 138, 139, 140, 141, 142

K

kindergarten, 22
knees, 28

L

landscape, 72
languages, 118
laws, 66, 114, 127, 128
lead, 12, 20, 21
leadership, 55, 117
learning, 22, 23, 39, 46, 56, 57, 73, 134, 138
learning process, 22
Lebanon, 57
Lee County, 77
legislation, 15, 114, 115, 127, 128, 130, 135
legs, 4, 27, 28, 144
leisure, 10
leisure time, 10
lens, 9, 32, 106
lesson plan, 57
lifetime, vii, 1, 2, 6, 54, 110
light, 5, 7, 10, 21, 35, 48, 50, 52, 60, 149
literacy, 23, 39
longevity, 76, 118
Louisiana, 126
lymph, 4
lymph node, 4

M

magazines, 23, 37, 139
magnesium, 39
magnetic declination, 70
magnetic field, 70
majority, ix, 4, 10, 19, 22, 107, 110
malignancy, 56
malignant melanoma, 31, 32, 34, 40, 54, 106
management, 34
marketing, 36
Marshall Islands, 121
Marx, 39
Maryland, 126
materials, ix, xi, 2, 7, 56, 57, 65, 91, 103, 108, 109, 115, 123, 124, 125, 128, 130, 135
matter, 60
measurement(s), 22, 51, 69, 70, 83, 98
media, 21, 23, 124, 139
medical, 3, 8, 29, 75, 78
medicine, 3, 15, 116
melanin, 6, 53

melanoma, vii, 1, 2, 3, 4, 6, 7, 9, 10, 30, 31, 32, 33, 34, 35, 36, 38, 44, 45, 54, 56, 74, 79, 80, 106, 110, 122, 125, 140, 142, 149
mental health, 13
meridian, 83
messages, 20, 21, 23, 137
metabolism, 53
metropolitan areas, 120
Mexico, 121
minors, 114, 127, 135
mission, 18, 55, 56, 131
misuse, 37
model trees, 90
models, 20, 23, 24, 39, 90
modifications, 76
mole, 7
Montana, 127
morbidity, ix, 11, 107
mortality, ix, 2, 4, 5, 11, 32, 107, 120, 121
mortality rate, 2, 4, 5, 32
MR, 37
multimedia, 56
museums, 111, 133, 136

N

National Center for Education Statistics (NCES), 122
National Comprehensive Cancer Control Program (NCCCP), ix, 107, 149
National Institutes of Health, 34, 45, 55
national policy, 13
Natural Resources Conservation Service, 65
networking, 66
New England, 149
New South Wales, 36, 39
NOAA, 49, 52
North America, 120
nurses, viii, 14, 16, 24, 25, 44, 115, 125, 135, 139, 140, 141
nursing, 3, 116
nutrition, 13, 39, 113, 117

O

obesity, 117, 130
officials, 46
opportunities, vii, viii, 1, 3, 6, 7, 14, 19, 21, 39, 43, 110, 111, 122, 124, 125, 129, 131, 133, 147, 150
oral health, 147
orbit, 86, 87
organize, 16, 129
organs, 4
outreach, 16, 80
oversight, 113, 117
ozone, 5, 21, 48, 50, 106
ozone layer, 5, 48, 50, 106

P

Pacific, 120
parallel, 83
parental consent, 141
parents, 3, 11, 15, 16, 18, 19, 23, 25, 26, 27, 33, 37, 41, 46, 47, 55, 59, 67, 75, 78, 79, 115, 125, 136, 138, 139, 140
participants, 73, 129, 141
pathogenesis, 31, 149
pediatrics, viii, 2
peer influence, 23
per capita income, 74, 77
permission, 15, 18, 25, 94, 96, 139
pharmaceutical, 19
phosphorus, 39
photosynthesis, 52
physical activity, 11, 31, 46, 113, 117, 133, 148
physical education, 13, 14, 17, 21, 45, 75, 78, 92, 95, 113
physical environment, ix, 16, 44, 136
physicians, 35
pigmentation, 53
pilot study, 33, 41
plants, 63, 64, 65, 66
PM, 38, 52

policy, ix, x, 13, 15, 16, 17, 18, 19, 24, 26, 35, 39, 45, 74, 81, 103, 108, 109, 110, 115, 117, 119, 127, 128, 130, 131, 133, 134, 135, 140, 147, 150
policy initiative, 17
policy issues, x, 109, 119, 127
policy options, 17
policymakers, 3
polycarbonate, 60
pools, 119, 136
population, 5, 10, 15, 32, 37, 38, 74, 77, 106
poverty, 74, 77
preadolescents, 11
precipitation, 93, 95, 96
preparation, 37
President, 138
primary school, 40, 110, 131
principles, 13
professional development, viii, ix, 2, 13, 14, 24, 26, 44, 108, 139
professionals, viii, 3, 20, 25, 44, 140, 150
profit, 56, 73, 80
progress reports, 141
project, 32, 40, 46, 47, 59, 64, 67, 72, 75, 76, 81, 103, 106, 125
PST, 49
psychology, 73
public health, viii, 2, 3, 11, 116, 129, 150
public schools, 74, 117
public service, 115
Puerto Rico, 57, 120

Q

quality control, 36
Queensland, 31, 39
query, 91
questionnaire, 150

R

radiation, vii, viii, 1, 2, 4, 5, 7, 8, 9, 10, 11, 12, 14, 15, 23, 31, 32, 34, 35, 36, 41, 43, 44, 45, 47, 48, 49, 50, 51, 52, 53, 54, 60, 61, 62, 69, 71, 75, 76, 78, 86, 88, 98, 101, 106, 110, 134, 149
rainfall, 64
RE, 39
reactions, 37
recognition, 20
recommendations, viii, x, xi, 3, 9, 13, 15, 27, 33, 43, 68, 71, 91, 92, 101, 102, 103, 109, 119, 149
recovery, 74
recreation, 3, 16, 19, 20, 23, 24, 27, 40, 41, 111, 117, 137
recreational, 36, 117
reflectivity, 101
registries, 4, 44, 120
regulations, 113, 127
rehabilitation, ix, 107
reintroduction, 48, 84
relatives, 7
relevance, 13, 58
repair, 7
reputation, 130
requirements, 12, 15, 72, 79
resistance, 78
resolution, 116, 135
resource allocation, 16
response, 32, 52, 85, 106
restrictions, 15, 64, 127
rewards, 64
RH, 37
rickets, 12, 106
risk(s), vii, viii, 1, 2, 3, 4, 5, 6, 7, 10, 11, 13, 16, 21, 26, 32, 33, 34, 35, 36, 37, 38, 41, 43, 46, 50, 51, 54, 56, 60, 71, 78, 88, 100, 106, 110, 121, 132, 143, 150
risk factors, 21, 33, 34, 38, 56, 106, 143
root(s), 63
rules, 15, 17, 128

S

school activities, 13, 18, 110, 113, 139
school community, 46, 73, 91, 101, 102

school grounds, ix, 18, 44, 45, 46, 51, 58, 59, 61, 63, 67, 68, 69, 70, 71, 73, 75, 91, 92, 93, 94, 95, 96, 97, 98, 99, 100, 101
school psychology, 3
science, 15, 19, 64, 65, 113, 123, 125
scientific knowledge, 57
scope, 76
SEA, 114
seasonal changes, 48, 71, 84
secondary schools, 39, 77
seed, 106
sensitivity, 53
service provider, 3
services, 13, 14, 57, 58, 78, 96, 110, 113
sexuality, 147
shape, 89
showing, 48, 121
shrubs, 46, 62, 63, 64, 65, 102
signs, 17, 20
skill acquisition, 22
skin cancer risks, vii, viii, 2
skin diseases, 33, 35
soccer, 41, 69
social environment, viii, 14, 19, 20, 26, 43, 135
social learning, 21
social norms, 19, 20, 135
software, 90, 100
solar collectors, 90
solution, 47, 101, 102
solvents, 50
South Africa, 106
South Dakota, 127
specialists, viii, 2, 3, 16, 25, 62, 140
species, 63, 65, 70, 72, 99
specifications, 75
sports events, 136
squamous cell, 3, 4, 5, 6, 9, 27, 35, 44, 54, 109, 149
squamous cell carcinoma, 3, 4, 5, 6, 9, 27, 35, 54
SS, 32
staff development, 16, 143, 147, 148
stakeholder groups, 67, 68, 71, 92
stakeholders, 46, 72, 93, 113, 118, 129
state laws, 114, 115
statistics, 31, 55, 73, 120, 149
steel, 46, 75, 79
structure, 59, 60, 61, 62, 63, 75, 77, 78, 81, 83, 94, 95, 96, 97, 100, 101, 103, 115, 124
sunburn, 6, 8, 11, 20, 25, 32, 33, 37, 38, 45, 52, 55, 106, 110, 144, 146, 148
supplementation, 12, 36, 39
suppression, 5, 36
surveillance, xi, 109, 120, 122, 130, 142, 143, 150
survival, 64
survivors, 125
susceptibility, 11, 52
sustainability, 110, 118
symptoms, 53
synthesis, 12, 52, 53

T

target, 121, 122, 123, 124
Task Force, 8, 9, 131, 149
teaching strategies, 24
team members, 48, 72
teams, 17, 47, 48, 68, 73, 83, 102, 117, 125, 135, 140
technical assistance, 25, 123, 135, 141
technical support, ix, 107
techniques, 21, 70, 73
teens, 140
temperature, 46, 63, 74, 76, 106
term plans, 68
territory, ix, x, xi, 107, 108, 109, 111, 113, 119, 120, 123, 124, 128, 133, 135, 136, 137, 138, 139, 140, 141, 142
testing, 10
textiles, 36
the National Oceanic and Atmospheric Administration's, 51
thoughts, 131
threats, 58, 78, 129, 131, 150
time frame, 57
tobacco, 31, 117, 130
toddlers, 12

trade, 57
training, 2, 24, 25, 26, 55, 115, 135, 140, 141
training programs, 2
transmission, 9, 18, 23
treatment, ix, 55, 107
trial, 9, 36, 41
tribal organization, ix, 107

U

U.S. Department of Agriculture, 65
United, vii, 1, 2, 3, 4, 9, 10, 19, 23, 32, 34, 40, 44, 55, 57, 63, 65, 74, 77, 79, 80, 84, 87, 102, 106, 115, 120, 121, 125, 151
United Nations, 106
United Nations Development Program, 106
United States, vii, 1, 2, 3, 4, 9, 10, 19, 23, 32, 34, 40, 44, 55, 57, 63, 65, 74, 77, 79, 80, 84, 87, 102, 115, 120, 121, 125, 151
universities, 116
urban, 65, 66
US Department of Health and Human Services, 31, 34
USA, 119
USDA, 63, 64, 65
UV exposure, vii, 1, 4, 6, 9, 10, 12, 21, 26, 131, 148
UV light, 3, 110
UV radiation, vii, 1, 4, 5, 6, 7, 8, 9, 10, 12, 14, 17, 21, 22, 26, 35, 44, 45, 47, 49, 50, 51, 52, 53, 54, 55, 60, 61, 62, 63, 71, 76, 80, 81, 88, 91, 100, 101, 102, 110, 128

V

vandalism, 71, 94, 96, 97
varieties, 63
vegetation, 46, 58, 63, 64, 70, 72, 102
vision(s), 75, 131
vitamin D, 12, 39, 52, 53, 106
vitamin D deficiency, 106
voluntary organizations, 29
Volunteers, 72

W

Wales, 36
Washington, 30, 31, 34, 39, 56, 66, 70
water, 7, 10, 28, 50, 51, 64, 119
wear, 3, 17, 28, 121, 136, 144, 145
web, 49, 73, 91, 114, 116, 117, 119, 120, 123, 127, 129
web pages, 114, 116, 117, 119, 123, 127, 129
well-being, 113
wellness, 113
Western Australia, 33, 149
wildlife, 64, 101, 102
windstorms, 76
Wisconsin, 126
wood, 106
workers, 55
World Health Organization, 51
worldwide, 23, 66

Y

yield, 2, 19, 110, 142
young adults, 2, 3, 55
young people, ix, x, 31, 108, 109, 110, 111, 113, 114, 117, 118, 121, 122, 123, 131, 132, 133, 135, 143, 148